The Quiet Killer

Emphysema / Chronic Obstructive Pulmonary Disease

Edited by
Hannah L. Hedrick
Austin H. Kutscher
and the editors of the
American Institute of Life-Threatening Illness and Loss

The Scarecrow Press, Inc.
Lanham, Maryland, and London
2002

SCARECROW PRESS, INC.

Published in the United States of America
by Scarecrow Press, Inc.
4720 Boston Way, Lanham, Maryland 20706
www.scarecrowpress.com

4 Pleydell Gardens, Folkestone
Kent CT20 2DN, England

British Library Cataloguing-in-Publication Information Available

Library of Congress Cataloging-in-Publication Data

The quiet killer : emphysema–chronic obstructive pulmonary disease / edited by
Hannah L. Hedrick, Austin H. Kutscher, and the editors of the American Institute
of Life-Threatening Illness and Loss.
    p. ; cm.
   Includes bibliographical references.
   ISBN 0-8108-4173-8 (cloth : alk. paper)
   1. Emphysema, Pulmonary–Patients–Care. 2. Lungs–Diseases, Obstructive–Patients–
Care. 3. Terminal care. I. Title: Emphysema–chronic obstructive pulmonary disease.
II. Hedrick, Hannah L. III. Kutscher, Austin H. IV. American Institute of Life-
Threatening Illness and Loss.
   [DNLM: 1. Pulmonary Emphysema–therapy. 2. Lung Diseases, Obstructive–
therapy. 3. Palliative Care. 4. Terminal Care. WF 648 Q605 2002]
RC776.O3 Q54 2002
616.2'4–dc21   2001054930

♾™ The paper used in this publication meets the minimum requirements of
American National Standard for Information Sciences—Permanence of
Paper for Printed Library Materials, ANSI/NISO Z39.48-1992.
Manufactured in the United States of America.

This volume is dedicated to
the life and loving benefactions of
Beatrice Snyder.

Contents

Contents

Preface

Thomas L. Petty, MD

Emphysema/Chronic Obstructive Pulmonary Disease (COPD) is this nation's most rapidly growing health problem. Today COPD/emphysema is the fourth most common cause of death, with approximately 110,000 patients reaching the end of their lives each year. Although much has been done to improve the length and the quality of life in people with COPD/emphysema, including ambulatory oxygen and pulmonary rehabilitation, the diseases continue to progress.

It is important that patients, health care providers, the public, and governmental agencies understand the problems faced by patients with advanced stages of COPD/emphysema. Modern science has extended both the length and the quality of life for most sufferers of COPD; many live into their 70s or 80s. Ambulatory oxygen therapy and techniques of pulmonary rehabilitation are established as the standard of care for patients who want to try to pursue full activities of daily living and a zestful transition into the aging, and ultimately the dying, process.

Death should not be viewed as the enemy. Death is a normal consequence of having lived. The enemy is loneliness, fear, anxiety, depression, and sorrow. These powerful limiting states can be mitigated by understanding that, as death becomes near, chronic carbon dioxide retention begins to occur. The slow building of carbon dioxide is often soothing. This is compensated by balancing metabolic factors that usually keep the acid activity of the blood in the normal or near normal range, until energy failure occurs in all the tissues of the body. When the brain, lungs, heart, kidneys, and other vital organs fail, death occurs. Death should be likened to a long and restful sleep. What lies beyond should be considered an adventure, very much like being born. I hope that we will all look forward to this new journey, which itself represents an exciting transition of the human spirit.

The American Institute of Life-Threatening Illness and Loss sponsored its first symposium on dealing with the advanced stages of COPD in 1999, after several years of meetings and communication with physician professional associations, professional associations of related health professions, and consumer and self-help groups. The outcomes of the 1999 meeting are reflected in this publication, which served as background information for the September 2000 Strategic Planning Colloquium for a Composite COPD/Emphysema Program, to include establishing a national COPD/emphysema association, journal, and colloquium series. If you are interested in participating in this initiative, please contact Dr. Austin H. Kutscher, president, The American Institute of Life-Threatening Illness and Loss.

Acknowledgments

The editors wish to express their appreciation for the support and encouragement of The American Institute of Life-Threatening Illness and Loss, a division of the Foundation of Thanatology, in the preparation of this volume. The field of thanatology encompasses scientific and humanistic inquiries and the application of the knowledge derived therefrom to the medical and psychological aspects of serious and life-threatening illness.

We wish to thank Mary Franco for her scrupulously detailed editing and intelligent queries, which greatly strengthened the chapters. The editing and desktop publishing contributions of Mary O'Leary also exceeded our expectations.

The editors and The American Institute also wish to express their deep appreciation for the generous support of the Beatrice Snyder Foundation and the Gloria and Louis Flanzer Philanthropic Fund in the preparation and publication of this volume.

Finally, The American Institute wishes to express its deepest appreciation for the very generous donation from the National Emphysema Foundation on behalf of the efforts of The American Institute, which has enabled the publication of this volume.

General Editors

Hannah L. Hedrick, PhD
Director, Division of Medical Education Products,
Editor, AMA's *Cultural Competence Compendium*,
American Medical Association, Chicago, Illinois

Dr. Austin H. Kutscher
President, The American Institute of Life-Threatening
Illness and Loss; Department of Psychiatry, College
of Physicians and Surgeons, Columbia University,
New York, New York

Contributing Editors

Paul Fairman, MD, FACP, FCCP
Professor of Medicine, Virginia Commonwealth
University, Medical College of Virginia,
Pulmonary and Critical Care, Richmond, Virginia

Thomas D. Whitman
E.F.F.O.R.T.S. (Emphysema Foundation for
Our Right to Survive), Palm Bay, Florida

Sreedhar Nair, MD
Chairman and Medical Director, National
Emphysema Foundation, Norwalk, Connecticut

John Leaman
President and Coordinator, Asthma/Emphysema
Self-Help Group, New York, New York

Barbara Rogers
Director of Breethezy™, New York, New York

Byron M. Thomashow, MD
Professor of Clinical Medicine, College of Physicians
and Surgeons, Columbia University; Medical Director,
Lung Failure Center, Columbia-Presbyterian Medical
Center, New York, New York

Contributors

Janet L. Abrahm, MD, FACP
Associate Professor of Medicine,
University of Pennsylvania School of Medicine,
Philadelphia, Pennsylvania

Hormoz Ashtyani, MD
Medical Director, The Breath and Lung Institute,
Hackensack University Medical Center,
Hackensack, New Jersey

Diane M. Biskobing, MD
Assistant Professor, Division of Endocrinology,
Virginia Commonwealth University,
Richmond, Virginia

Anne H. Boyle, RN, PhD
Pulmonary Nurse Practitioner,
McGuire Veterans Administration Medical Center,
Richmond, Virginia

Sandra K. Brandley, CRT
Executive Director, Alpha 1 Association,
Minneapolis, Minnesota

Christine A. Cannon, RN, PhD
Associate Professor of Nursing, College of Health
and Nursing Sciences, University of Delaware,
Wilmington, Delaware

Mike Chaney, RRT
Adjunct Instructor, Respiratory Care Project,
Cincinnati State Technical and Community College,
Cincinnati, Ohio

Kevin R. Cooper, MD
Professor of Medicine, Medical College of Virginia,
Richmond, Virginia

Paul Fairman, MD, FACP, FCCP
Professor of Medicine, Virginia Commonwealth
University, Medical College of Virginia,
Pulmonary and Critical Care, Richmond, Virginia

Joseph F. Fennelly, MD
Private Practice (Internal Medicine),
Madison, New Jersey

Kristin Fless, MD
Fellow, Pulmonary and Critical Care Medicine,
University of Medicine and Dentistry of New Jersey,
Newark, New Jersey

Harold Haley, MD
Emeritus Professor of Clinical Surgery,
Baylor College of Medicine, Houston, Texas

Hannah L. Hedrick, PhD
Director, Division of Medical Education Products,
Editor, AMA's *Cultural Competence Compendium*,
American Medical Association, Chicago, Illinois

Daryl Holtz Isenberg, PhD
President, Illinois Self-Help Coalition, Chicago, Illinois

Phyllis Krug, RPT, MS, CCS
Certified Pulmonary Cardiopulmonary Specialist;
Rehabilitation Consultant and President, Lung Life, Inc.,
Teaneck, New Jersey

Debra Lierl, MEd, RRT
Program Chair (Respiratory Care), Program Director
(Emergency Medical Services), Cincinnati State Technical and Community College, Cincinnati, Ohio

Richard W. Light, MD
Director, Pulmonary Diseases, St. Thomas Hospital,
Nashville, Tennessee

Dianne L. Locke, RN, MN, CS
Pulmonary Nurse Practitioner, McGuire Veterans
Administration Medical Center, Richmond, Virginia

Sreedhar Nair, MD
Chairman and Medical Director, National Emphysema
Foundation, Norwalk, Connecticut

Phil Petersen
Author of *Good If Not Great Living with Lung Disease*.
Raven Publishers, Inc., Charlotte, North Carolina

Barbara Ann Phillips, MD, MSPh, FCCP
Professor of Pulmonary and Critical Care Medicine,
Pulmonary Division, University of Kentucky-Chandler
Medical Center, Lexington, Kentucky

Mary Pat Raimondi, MA
Research Assistant, Milestone Group,
St. Paul, Minnesota

Barbara Rogers
Director of Breethezy™, New York, New York

Larry L. Schulman, MD
Associate Professor of Clinical Medicine, College of
Physicians and Surgeons, Columbia University; Medical
Director of Lung Transplants, Columbia-Presbyterian
Medical Center, New York, New York

Helen M. Sorenson, RRT
Director of Clinical Education, Respiratory
Care Program, Metropolitan Community College,
Omaha, Nebraska

Julie Swanson
Member of Board of Directors, Alpha 1 Association,
Olathe, Kansas

Byron M. Thomashow, MD
Professor of Clinical Medicine, College of
Physicians and Surgeons, Columbia University;
Medical Director, Lung Failure Center, Columbia-
Presbyterian Medical Center, New York, New York

Thomas D. Whitman
E.F.F.O.R.T.S. (Emphysema Foundation for
Our Right to Survive), Palm Bay, Florida

Victoria D. Weisfeld
Senior Communications Officer, Robert Wood
Johnson Foundation, Chicago, Illinois

Introduction

In May 1987, the *Journal of Allied Health* published my article on "Allied Health Professionals and Patients with Life-Threatening Illness: A Holy Alliance." The article reported rather extensively on my first experience a month earlier with a symposium sponsored by the Foundation of Thanatology (The American Institute of Life-Threatening Illness and Loss was created later). The article described the goals of the symposium:

- Assess the roles and contributions of allied health personnel in the continuum of care provided to patients with life-threatening illness and to their families.
- Increase the ability of allied health professionals to plan, implement, and evaluate curricula in psychosocial aspects of patient care (especially those in advanced disease states).
- Promote the effectiveness of patient and family support systems.

I was struck by the sincere efforts of Dr. Austin "Bill" H. Kutscher, president of the Foundation of Thanatology, in bringing together more than fifty-five speakers from broadly diverse backgrounds: allied health professionals, educators, and researchers; suicidologists; psychosocial professionals; bereavement counselors; gerontologists; pet therapists; and self-help and other consumer groups. In my article, I commented that "one of the greatest benefits of the symposium was the opportunity to interact with individuals who shared a common commitment to exploring the ways in which allied health professionals can work with the patient, family, and community to improve the care and treatment of persons with life-threatening illness."

Since 1987, I have learned a lot about the Foundation of Thanatology and its more recently created division, The American Institute of Life-Threatening Illness and Loss, and my respect for and appreciation of Bill Kutscher's work has increased with each year. I especially appreciate the inclusive approach to presenters and participants, which usually include professionals, educators, and researchers from multiple medical professions, from various areas of nursing, and from dozens of other health-related areas. And programs almost always include a number of patient perspectives, either as individuals or as spokespersons for member or professionally led self-help groups.

I did not need to be told that the Foundation of Thanatology was the first organization devoted to improving care related to advanced disease states in multiple illnesses to conduct national, multidisciplinary, multiprofessional meetings that also included patient perspectives and medical/nursing education insights. I had been promoting such inclusion for more than two decades, both professionally (as an employee of the American Medical Association's Medical Education Group) and personally (as an advocate of people with disabilities and of self-help groups), only to be met with resistance, usually on the part of professionals. By the time then-Surgeon General C. Everett Koop, MD, sponsored the Surgeon General's Workshop on Self-Help and Public Health in 1987, Bill had been bringing professionals and consumers together for more than two decades. The Foundation of Thanatology and the AMA picked up the ball two years later by sponsoring the national symposium on "The Impact of Life-Threatening Conditions: Self-Help Groups and Health Care Providers in Partnership" (Chicago 1989), which led to the book *Self-Help: Concepts and Applications* (Charles Press 1992). Articles from this book, including the foreword by Dr. Koop, are frequently quoted in self-help literature.

The Foundation of Thanatology was incorporated and chartered by the Board of Regents of the University of the State of New York in 1967 as a public, tax-exempt educational and scientific organization. Based mainly at Columbia-Presbyterian Medical Center, the Foundation (and later The American Institute) has organized approximately 150 symposia and published nearly as many volumes focusing on medical education and quality of life aspects of diseases having multiple etiologies. These symposia have contributed significantly to the literature related to life-threatening illness and end-of-life care.

It is good to remind ourselves that while major national initiatives, such as the Robert Wood Johnson Foundation's Last Acts project and programs sponsored by the Project on Death in America, Americans for Better Care of the Dying, Partnership for Caring, and similar groups, deserve tremendous credit for improving the quality of end-of-life care, many of these efforts build on the 30-year track record of the Foundation of Thanatology and The American Institute of Life-Threatening Illness and Loss.

The present volume is the most recent in the Foundation of Thanatology/American Institute's long lineup. It is closely aligned with American Institute symposia on "orphan" diseases with multiple etiologies sponsored by many of the same organizations during the past four years, beginning in 1997 with "Non-Cancer Life-Threatening Diseases and Their End-of-Life Care Components." The articles in this volume both capture the content of the 1999 symposium on "Advanced Chronic Obstructive Pulmonary Disease" and set the stage for the "Strategic Planning Colloquium for a Composite COPD/Emphysema Program," held September 2000 at Columbia-Presbyterian Medical Center in New York City.

The 1999 symposium established an ambitious agenda of considering a composite COPD program, to be administered by The American Institute. Various committees and individuals working diligently during the past several years have established a program for moving forward with organizing a national COPD association, establishing a national COPD journal, and developing a series of colloquia to address unmet needs related to advanced COPD/emphysema.

If you are interested in participating in or receiving information about this project, please contact Dr. Austin Kutscher at 718/601-4453 or fax him at 718/549-7219. You will be in good company.

Hannah L. Hedrick, PhD
Director, Medical Education Products
American Medical Association

Part I

Managing Advanced-Stage COPD/Emphysema

1

Managing Dyspnea

Richard W. Light, MD

One of the most disturbing symptoms that patients with chronic obstructive pulmonary disease (COPD) have is dyspnea. Dyspnea by definition is discomfort experienced during breathing. The exercise tolerance of most patients with COPD is limited by dyspnea. As the disease progresses, the dyspnea becomes more pronounced with less activity and, eventually, in the terminal phase, the patient becomes dyspneic at rest. It is believed that dyspnea for the COPD patient is analogous to pain for the cancer patient. The presence of severe dyspnea makes the COPD patient miserable. Caregivers should attempt to alleviate the dyspnea.

Why do COPD patients develop dyspnea? In general, development is related to three factors: (1) the maximal breathing capacity of the patient, (2) the actual breathing requirement of the patient, and (3) the sensitivity of the dyspnea center. This relationship can be expressed by the following equation:

EQUATION 1

dyspnea = actual ventilation x sensitivity of dyspnea sensor

Ventilatory Capacity

The degree of dyspnea that a patient experiences is not closely related to the level of pulmonary function. In general, the correlation coefficient between any measure of pulmonary function and the exercise tolerance is about 0.60, which indicates that only about 36% of the variance in the exercise tolerance can be explained by the level of pulmonary dysfunction. The exercise tolerance of a group of patients with an FEV_1 of 1000 ml may vary as much as threefold.

There are several reasons for the variation in the exercise tolerance of patients with COPD. Some insight into the reasons for these variations can be attained by considering the factors that determine the ventilatory requirements for a given patient at rest or during exercise. In general, the carbon dioxide produced by the body needs to be eliminated with ventilation. The amount of carbon dioxide eliminated is given by the following equation:

EQUATION 2

$$Vco_2 = V_E \times Paco_2/760 \times (1 - V_D/V_T)$$

in which Vco_2 is the production of carbon dioxide, V_E is the minute ventilation, V_D is the dead space ventilation per breath, and V_T is the tidal volume. Equation 1 can be rewritten in the following manner to demonstrate the factors upon which the V_E depends:

EQUATION 3

$$V_E = Vco_2 / [Paco_2/760 \times (1 - V_D/V_T)]$$

One primary factor determining the level of ventilation is the Vco_2. From Equation 3 it can be seen that the higher the Vco_2, the higher the ventilatory requirement. Since the Vco_2 is proportional to the intensity of the exercise, the higher the intensity of the exercise the greater the ventilatory requirement. Another key factor is the $Paco_2$. The higher the $Paco_2$, the lower the ventilatory requirement. If the $Paco_2$ increases from 40 to 80 mm Hg, then the required ventilation is halved at any level of Vco_2. Another key factor is the percentage of wasted ventilation (V_D/V_T). The higher the percentage of wasted ventilation, the higher the V_E for a given Vco_2. In patients with COPD, about 40% of the ventilation is wasted, but there is much interindividual variation.

Another important factor in determining the level of dyspnea is the relationship between the degree of dyspnea and the ratio of the actual ventilation to the patient's ventilatory capacity. Some patients may become very dyspneic if the ratio is 40%; others may not become dyspneic until the relationship exceeds 80%. This sensitivity is reflected in the classic descriptions of the "pink puffer" and the "blue bloater." Although the two individuals have a similar FEV_1, the pink puffer (with predominantly emphysema) is dyspneic at rest and unable to perform much exercise although he is well oxygenated. In contrast, the blue bloater does not feel dyspneic at rest or with mild exercise but is hypoxemic with carbon dioxide retention. The pink puffer's brain is much more sensitive to a given level of ventilation than is the blue bloater's.

How Do We Decrease Dyspnea?

In general, there are three different ways that the level of dyspnea can be decreased at a given Vco_2: (1) increase the ventilatory capabilities of the patient, (2) decrease the patient's ventilatory requirements, and (3) alter the relationship between the degree of dyspnea and the ratio of the actual ventilation to the ventilatory capacity.

Increasing the Ventilatory Capabilities

Most efforts by physicians taking care of patients with advanced COPD are aimed at improving the ventilatory capabilities. The administration of bronchodilators, such as the beta adrenergic compounds, anticholinergics and theophylline, are directed toward improving patients' ventilatory capabilities. Corticosteroids, either inhaled or oral, are also given with the hope of improving such capabilities. However, most research concerning these agents deals with the effects they had on pulmonary function rather than on dyspnea. Nevertheless, since the maximal minute ventilation of patients with COPD is approximately 37 times their FEV_1, an improvement in the FEV_1 would be expected to decrease the level of dyspnea at a given VCO_2.

Surgery, either lung-volume reduction or lung transplantation, has been advocated as a means to improve lung function. While there is no doubt that either of these surgical maneuvers will improve lung function, they are not appropriate for many patients with advanced COPD. Nevertheless, they should be considered for all such patients.

Decreasing the Ventilatory Requirements

Most patients with advanced COPD decrease their ventilatory requirements by decreasing their exercise. However, there are other means to decrease these requirements. The simplest means by which the ventilatory requirements can be decreased is if the $PaCO_2$ increases. This is most commonly accomplished via the administration of supplemental oxygen, but it can also be accomplished via the administration of opiates or benzodiazepams.

Altering the Perception of Dyspnea

The three most common ways to alter the perception of dyspnea are to administer oxygen, opiates, or benzodiazepams.

Administering Oxygen

Supplemental oxygen is usually administered to correct hypoxemia. Indeed, hypoxemia is the only indication that Medicare will acknowledge for reimbursement for chronic oxygen therapy. Hypoxemia tends to exacerbate dyspnea for two reasons. First, the presence of hypoxemia will stimulate ventilation. Accordingly, as seen from Equation 1, dyspnea will be increased because of the increased ventilation. Second, at a given level of ventilation, dyspnea is greater if there is hypoxemia because the brain's sensor for dyspnea is more sensitive.

However, supplemental oxygen can also reduce dyspnea even if the patient does not meet published criteria for supplemental oxygen. The primary mechanism by which supplemental oxygen decreases the ventilatory requirement is due to its effect on the $PaCO_2$. The average increase in the

5

$PaCO_2$ when supplemental oxygen is administered chronically is about 10% (Berry et al 1993). From Equation 3, it can be seen that if the $PaCO_2$ increases by 10%, the ventilation should decrease by 10% and dyspnea should decrease. In one study, the resting minute ventilation decreased from 12.3 $\pm$ 0.46 to 11.6 $\pm$ 0.47 L/min when 14 COPD patients with a mean SaO_2 over 90% were given supplemental oxygen via nasal cannula at 2L/min (Berry et al). In the same study, the administration of supplemental oxygen led to a significant decrease in the mouth occlusion pressure developed in the first 100 ms of inspiration (P0.1). The mouth occlusion pressure is thought to be an index of respiratory drive.

The best way to administer oxygen, if alleviation of dyspnea is the main goal, is transtracheally. The advantage of transtracheal oxygen as compared with oxygen administered nasally is that when oxygen is administered transracheally, it markedly decreases the inspired minute ventilation. In one study (Couser 1989), the mean resting inspired minute ventilation at rest decreased from 9.8 $\pm$ 2.3 to 5.8 $\pm$ 1.1 L/min when oxygen was administered transtracheally at 4 L/min. Indeed, if air rather than oxygen is administered transtracheally, the inspiratory ventilation will also decrease significantly. In effect, when oxygen is administered transtracheally, the inspiratory ventilation of the patient decreases and the decrease is approximately equal to the amount of air delivered transtracheally. In other words, the transtracheal air functions as a partial ventilator. The primary problem with transtracheal ventilation at the present time is related to technical problems with the placement and maintenance of the transtracheal catheter.

Administering Opiates

For the past 50 years there has been hesitancy on the part of the medical community to administer opiates to dyspneic patients with advanced COPD because of the fear that use in this situation could lead to marked increases in the $PaCO_2$, respiratory acidosis, coma, and even death. However, it should be noted that opiates are quite effective in alleviating dyspnea.

Woodcock and associates generated interest in the use of opiates in patients with COPD in the early 1980s, when they demonstrated that the acute administration of dihydrocodeine, 1 mg/kg, to 12 patients with COPD (mean FEV = 0.73 L) significantly reduced the patients' dyspnea during exercise and increased the exercise tolerance (Woodcock et al 1982). It was subsequently demonstrated in 13 patients with a mean FEV_1 of 0.90 that the administration of 0.8 mg/kg morphine orally resulted in a nearly 20% increase in the maximum workload tolerated (Light et al 1989). The morphine appeared to increase the exercise tolerance by two different mechanisms. First, the morphine acted as a ventilatory depressant such that the $PaCO_2$ increased by about 10% and thus the ventilatory requirements were decreased by about 10%. Second, the morphine decreased the level of dyspnea associated with each level of ventilation. Indeed the ventilation at the maximal workload was approximately 10% greater after morphine than it was after placebo. Unfortunately, the dose of morphine used in this study (0.8 mg/kg) induced significant drowsiness.

It was later demonstrated that similar improvements could be obtained in the exercise tolerance and the level of dyspnea when the combination of morphine, 30 mg, and Phenergan, 25 mg, was acutely administered orally (Light et al 1996). With the combination of morphine and Phenergan, the mental status was not significantly affected. A lower dose of morphine (30 mg) did not significantly affect the exercise tolerance or reduce the dyspnea.

The more chronic use of opiates for the relief of dyspnea has not been well studied. Woodcock and colleagues performed a double-blind placebo-controlled crossover study comparing dihydrocodeine, 30 and 60 mg 3 times a day, and placebo each for 2 weeks. The patients had a mean FEV_1 of 0.75 and a mean $PaCO_2$ of 33.2 mm Hg. The results of this study were discouraging. Five of the 16 patients withdrew because of nausea and vomiting after taking dihydrocodeine. Of the 11 patients who completed the study, two were constipated and drowsy while taking dihydrocodeine and two had symptoms of opiate withdrawal after the 60 mg dose was stopped. However, there was a marked improvement in subjective disability when the 30 mg dose was given instead of the higher dose.

A later study by the same group (Johnson et al 1983) compared 1-week trials of dihydrocodeine, 15 mg, or placebo 30 minutes before exercise as required up to three times daily. In this study, there appeared to be significant benefit from the dihydrocodeine, since at the end of the treatment periods, the maximum distance patients walked was 16.5% higher and the breathlessness was 11.8% less than at equivalent distances while the patients were not receiving dihydrocodeine.

In a study done several years ago, patients received 30 mg of a sustained release morphine (MS-Contin) plus 25 mg Phenergan or placebo twice a day each for 2 weeks, separated by a 2-week washout (Light et al 1992). Some patients could not tolerate the active drugs because of constipation or mental cloudiness. If the frequency of the medications were reduced to once a day, the mental complaints became less troublesome. In general, the exercise tolerance and the degree of dyspnea were improved in the patients while they were receiving the active medications. At the end of the 6-week study period, the patients were given the option of continuing to take the active medications. Sleep studies showed that there was no more desaturation while the patients were receiving the active medications than while they were receiving placebo.

In the chronic study, eight patients continued the combination of MS Contin, 30 mg, and Phenergan, 25 mg, daily. Three of the patients continued on these medications for more than 2 years. One patient eventually had a lung transplant and stated that he would never have survived to receive his lung transplant if he had not been receiving the morphine-Phenergan combination. None of the patients appeared to develop tachyphylaxis for the opiates, and the dose was never increased above its original level in any of the patients. When the patients stopped the medications, there were no significant withdrawal symptoms.

A recent study in which patients received 10 to 20 mg sustained-release morphine showed no significant improvement compared with placebo (Poole et al 1998). It is unclear whether the explanation for the lack of effect was an insufficient dose of morphine or whether the concomitant use of Phenergan is important.

There have been very limited studies on the use of opiates for dyspnea in patients near the end of life. If dyspnea can be equated to pain in terms of decreasing the quality of life of these patients, consideration should be given to the use of opiates for the relief of dyspnea. In patients with cystic fibrosis, the use of opiates for end-of-life care has been shown to be effective in alleviating the debilitating dyspnea (Robinson et al 1997). In one series of 44 patients who died from cystic fibrosis, 11 patients (25%) had been receiving oral opiates for more than 3 months on a daily basis before their deaths. Opiates have also been shown to be of use in managing the dyspnea of patients with terminal cancer (Bruera et al 1990). It is recommended that all end-of-life patients with distressing dyspnea be given a trial of oral or parenteral opiates. It should be remembered, however, that hypoxemia can be exacerbated if opiates are given.

Although one report suggested that nebulized morphine was effective in relieving dyspnea in patients with lung disease (Young et al 1989), subsequent reports were unable to demonstrate any significant benefits with doses up to 30 mg (Beauford et al 1993, Noseda et al 1997).

Administering Benzodiazepines

There have been many anecdotal reports concerning the beneficial effects of benzodiazepines in the treatment of dyspneic patients with COPD. Mitchell-Heggs and coworkers (1980) kindled interest in the use of diazepam (Valium) in the treatment of the dyspneic patient with advanced COPD. In an uncontrolled study, they reported that breathlessness was improved dramatically in four patients with severe COPD (mean FEV_1 = 700 ml).

However, subsequent controlled studies have failed to demonstrate any benefit from the chronic administration of benzodiazepines to patients with COPD. Woodcock and associates (1981) reported that the administration of 25 mg Valium daily for 2 weeks to 15 patients with COPD (mean FEV_1 = 730 ml) had no effect on breathlessness and noticeably reduced exercise tolerance, while producing considerable drowsiness. Eimer and coworkers (1985) reported that the administration of clorazepate, 7.5 mg, at bedtime, to five patients with advanced COPD in a double-blind crossover study resulted in no improvement in exercise tolerance, arterial blood gases, self-rated breathlessness, or anxiety scores. Last, Man and associates (1986) administered alprazolam, 0.5 mg two times a day for 1 week, to 24 patients in a placebo-controlled crossover study and reported that there was no change in exercise tolerance or subjective sensations of dyspnea, although the PaO_2 tended to decrease and the $PaCO_2$ tended to increase. Accordingly, benzodiazepines are not recommended for the treatment of dyspnea in patients with COPD.

References

Beauford, W, TT Saylor, DW Stansbury, K Avalos, and RW Light. 1993. Effects of nebulized morphine sulfate on the exercise tolerance of the ventilatory limited COPD patient. *Chest*. 104:175-178.

Berry, RB, CK Mahutte, JL Kirsch, and RW Light. 1993. Does the hypoxic ventilatory response predict the oxygen-induced falls in ventilation in COPD? *Chest*. 103:820-824.

Bruera, E, K Macmillan, J Pither, and RN MacDonald. 1990. Effects of morphine on the dyspnea of terminal cancer patients. *J Pain Symptom Mgmt*. 5:341-344.

Couser, JI Jr and BJ Make. 1989. Transtracheal oxygen decreases inspired minute ventilation. *Am Rev Respir Dis*. 139:727-631.

Eimer, M, T Cable, P Gal et al. 1985. Effects of Clorazepate on breathlessness and exercise tolerance in patients with chronic airflow obstruction. *J Fam Practioner*. 21:359-362.

Johnson, MA, AA Woodcock, and DM Geddes. 1983. Dihydrocodeine for breathlessness in "pink puffers." *Br Med J*. 286:675-677.

Light, RW, DW Stansbury, and JS Webster. 1996. Effect of 30 mg of morphine alone or with Promethazine or Prochlorperazine on the exercise capacity of patients with COPD. *Chest*. 109:975-981.

Light, RW, DW Stansbury, K Avalos, JA Despars, FS Vargas, RB Berry, and VS Sayre. 1992. A study comparing the effects of morphine-Phenergan and placebo on the exercise tolerance and mentation of ventilatory limited COPD patients. *Chest*. 102:117S.

Light, RW, JR Muro, R Sato, DW Stansbury, CE Fischer, and SE Brown. 1989. Effects of oral morphine on breathlessness and exercise tolerance in patients with chronic obstructive pulmonary disease. *Am Rev Respir Dis*. 139:126-133.

Man, GCW, K Hsu, and BJ Sproule. 1986. Effect of Alprazolam on exercise and dyspnea in patients with chronic obstructive pulmonary disease. *Chest*. 90:832-836.

Mitchell-Heggs, P, K Murphy, K Minty et al. 1980. Diazepam in the treatment of dyspnea in the "pink puffer" syndrome. *Quarterly J Med*. 49:9-20.

Noseda, A, JP Carpiaux, C Markstein, A Meyvaert, and V de Maertelaer. 1997. Disabling dyspnea in patients with advanced disease: lack of effect of nebulized morphine. *Eur Respir J*. 10:1079-1083.

Poole, PJ, AG Veale, and PN Black. 1998. The effect of sustained-release morphine on breathlessness and quality of life in severe chronic obstructive pulmonary disease. *Am J Respir Crit Care Med*. 157:1877-1880.

Robinson, Wm, S Ravilly, C Berde, and ME Wohl. 1997. End-of-life care in cystic fibrosis. *Pediatrics*. 100:205-209.

Woodcock, AA, ER Gross, and DM Geddes. 1981. Drug treatment of breathlessness: contrasting effects of Diazepam and Promethazine in pink puffers. *Br Med J.* 283:343-345.

Woodcock, AA, MA Johnson, and DM Geddes. 1982. Breathlessness, alcohol, and opiates. *N Engl J Med.* 306:1611-1616.

Young, IH, E Daviskas, and VA Keena. 1989. Effect of low dose nebulised morphine on exercise endurance in patients with chronic lung disease. *Thorax.* 44:387-390.

2

Nocturnal Ventilatory Support in Enhancing Rehabilitation Potential

Phyllis Krug, RPT, MS, CCS

Studies have shown that the average patient with chronic obstructive pulmonary disease (COPD) struggles with the limitations of shortness of breath for up to 10 years before seeking medical advice (Dudley et al 1973). The patient's lifestyle has usually undergone changes that include a reduction in physical as well as social activity. The progressive nature of the disease and its concomitant sensation of shortness of breath discourages activity and, along with that, thoughts of hope, encouragement, progress, or improvement. The patient's physical limitation is intimately connected with a depressed psychological profile (Miller 1971).

As the disease progresses and the values of the pulmonary function test deteriorate, so too do the values measuring respiratory muscle strength (maximal inspiratory and expiratory pressure) and respiratory muscle endurance (maximum volume ventilation). It is unclear how intimately the role of muscle weakness is connected to the disease progression itself and how improved respiratory muscle strength affects the course of COPD. However, research in pulmonary rehabilitation and respiratory muscle training show that these approaches improve the condition of patients with chronic lung disease, as evidenced by increases in respiratory muscle strength and exercise capacity. There is also decreased oxygen consumption, despite insignificant changes in lung volume or flow measures (Berry 1996, Breslin 1996).

Other studies evaluate the effectiveness of nocturnal ventilation in relieving the dyspnea associated with COPD. The population of patients with COPD requiring nocturnal ventilation can be identified as having a rising level of $PaCO_2$. The elevated levels of CO_2 have a role in the associated problem of respiratory muscle weakness. Respiratory muscle fatigue is a critical factor in the requirement of nocturnal ventilation, and recent literature raises the question of its role in COPD (Amer Assn for Respiratory Care 1997). Although inconsistent, data may reflect the course of the disease of COPD where the hypertrophied respiratory muscles present in the earlier stages are replaced by weak atrophied muscles that are the result of overuse and malnutrition. Respiratory muscle fatigue is measured by a patient's inability to generate 50% of his or her maximum volume ventilation, as well as the inability to generate 60% to 80% of his or her inspiratory and expiratory muscle pressures. Fatigue can also be identified clinically by the onset of paradoxical breathing associated with rapid shallow breathing.

Without focusing on the specifics of positive or negative ventilators, nocturnal ventilator support has been found to be effective in significant populations in increasing exercise capacity, decreasing dyspnea, and increasing respiratory muscle strength (Clini 1998). Research, however, has not yet evaluated and compared patients undergoing rehabilitation with those receiving nocturnal ventilation. Would the patients that benefit from nocturnal support also benefit from rehabilitation? Is it possible that by using nocturnal ventilation and experiencing the subsequent relief of the work of breathing, patients would then best be suited for a more aggressive pulmonary rehabilitation program? This chapter suggests that the use of nocturnal ventilation is a key to improvement and presents a perspective that I have found to be clinically successful and that warrants future research and integration into accepted treatment.

Physiological Effects of Lung Disease

The energy cost of breathing is about 5% to 10% of a person's total capacity. For the patient struggling with shortness of breath, the cost of breathing can rise up to 70% of their total work capacity. This means that the person with severe COPD is working as hard to breathe at rest as the marathon runner at the end of a 25-mile run. For some patients at this level of metabolic work, exercise programs may actually be counterproductive. The concept of nocturnal ventilation is to offer patients a good night's sleep, an opportunity to rest their muscles so that they can begin the next day fresh (Rochester et al 1979, Braun and Marino 1984). I have found that once a patient has slept well for a few months, the opportunity for rehabilitation expands. Prior to a patient reaching this level of rest, the effort required to sustain life is all consuming. Breathing at rest is a monumental effort; the patient is hardly in optimal condition to consider the concepts of exercise, changing body mechanics, energy efficiency, etc. Further approaches need to wait until physiological rest has been achieved, as measured by reduction in $PaCO_2$ and improvement in oxygenation.

Breathing begins in the neck and ends at the sacrum; it requires flexion and extension of the total spinal column. Any restriction in its total mobility will limit breathing capability (Frownfelter and Massery 1996). In addition to mobility of the joints and muscles, it is critical to also look at the internal organs. The breathing mechanism relies on pressure changes between the chest and abdominal cavity. Any changes in the position or function of an organ will affect this pressure gradient. Surgical scarring can create adhesions that limit the glide and ease of movement of the organs, thus increasing resistance and pressure. Significant scarring in the abdomen, therefore, can increase the load of resistance to breathing.

Many chest wall changes can occur as a result of lung disease. Various muscles may be overused or underused, resulting in inefficient muscle contraction. Optimal muscle efficiency requires that muscles go through a full excursion of shortening and lengthening. The tendency of upper respiratory muscles to shorten and overwork can be due to distortions that take place in the chest wall as a result of air trapping. The musculoskeletal and organ changes that occur in response to lung disease develop slowly over time. Patients rely on their pattern of breathing, and interventions to alter these dynamics are very difficult to provide. However, with the use of nocturnal ventilators and the opportunity to rest comes a new field for intervention.

The following discussion on treating patients using nocturnal ventilators is meant only as an introduction of possibilities. As awareness grows, many more possibilities will emerge.

Breathing Retraining on the Ventilator

Patients struggle so much to breathe and spend so much of their daily existence thinking about breathing, yet they often do not know where they breathe from or how deeply. Resting on the ventilator is an optimal time to work on kinesthetic awareness of movement of different parts of the chest wall, concentrating on the anterior/posterior movement, lateral expansion, and upper chest expansion. It is possible to use intention or thought to control air movement. Beginning with tactile information, patients can increase awareness of movement of the chest wall and learn to maintain that control even without the tactile information. Patients can be taught to breathe into a specific area of the lung or allow the machine to push air into a specific area of the lung. Because patients are not working when using the ventilator, they have the luxury of being able to feel the movement and increase their sense of control.

While on ventilator support, patients are better able to tolerate supine (flat) positions, and therapies often impossible to administer because of patient discomfort or shortness of breath can be conducted with breathing support. Treatment directed at sacrum and pelvic mobility allows a freedom of movement of the spinal column that can have dramatic effects on improving breathing capability. Often, patients will report a sense of increased breathing and ease of chest wall movement while receiving treatment to the pelvic girdle. Many patients who suffer from shortness of breath are unable to lie flat; therefore, their musculature and joints are always in a forward-flexed position. Ventilator support provides the added breathing support necessary for more position variations, thus allowing for more optimal spinal elongation. This becomes the groundwork for enhancing pelvic and thoracic mobilization, as well as improved cervical mobility. The use of this breathing support provides the opportunity to address total body movement, resulting in improved breathing capability, which in turn leads to improved breathing and mobility when off the ventilator. For many patients, this approach alone suffices to improve breathing and "distance-walked" capabilities prior to any endurance training program.

Because the total spine flexes and extends with respiration, any restrictions of the spinal column will limit ventilator ability. Injuries, new or old, from the cranium to the coccyx will form a restriction. It need not be an obvious limitation in breathing capability, but because breathing is something we do 24 hours a day, a small restriction in movement can become a major obstacle over time. Patients with COPD typically rely on upper respiratory muscles to breathe as the disease progresses. This usually happens because, as the air trapping progresses and the girth of the rib cage expands, the diaphragm is put at a mechanical disadvantage and can actually begin to function as an expiratory muscle. Over the years, the patient simply learns to rely on the upper respiratory muscles. This excessive workload strains the cervical musculature and first and second rib, as well as clavicle attachments. The shortening of these muscles can cause pain and even compression of the thoracic outlet. The musculature pulls on neighboring structures connecting to the temporomandibular joint, hyoid, thyroid, and cricoid cartilages. The shortening musculature adds to the discomfort and causes compression to the vasculature where a patient is already struggling to breathe, but patients feel insecure "letting go" of these muscles because they are their lifelines. However, when patients have adjusted to nocturnal ventilation both physically and psychologically, a new kind of security emerges. There is a place to go to breathe. Even more so, as the months progress and true rest occurs, there is a resurgence of energy and an ease of breathing while off the ventilator. It is at this time that breathing reorganization, or retraining, can take place. The retraining looks at the total body and for restrictions throughout. Improvement and ease of movement throughout the body will translate into ease of breathing. Sometimes breathing reeducation is not necessary because, with the increased overall mobility, the body finds its own improved breathing without instruction.

Endurance Training

Aerobic training is an endurance activity that changes the structure of muscle fibers, resulting in more efficient oxygen uptake and less shortness of breath. Literature is very specific about a concept called muscle specificity, which means that muscles that are trained or exercised are the muscles that will benefit from the physiological changes associated with aerobic training (Knuttgen 1979). Thus, training on a treadmill will improve the walking muscles and not provide any improvement to other muscle groups. Typically, patients with COPD have minimal thoracic and pelvic rotation and a very short stride length. If these patients are placed on a treadmill, they will retain the rigid chest wall, poor mobility, and short stride length. However, improvement can be seen by the fact that they will be able to walk further. Simply put, this population of patients with poor mobility will benefit from training on a treadmill by being able to inefficiently move a longer distance! And by addressing the poor mobility issues, endurance improves, prior to the use of any endurance equipment.

It is possible to walk with ventilator support on a treadmill; both volume and pressure ventilators have been effective in providing additional breathing assistance to help patients keep up with more aggressive exercise. Even when off ventilator support, muscles still receive exercise and patients have the benefit of their increased strength and endurance. Nocturnal ventilators can be modified to assist those patients who cannot undergo an aerobic training program because of shortness of breath. One patient who used a negative pressure ventilator found it increasingly difficult to get off the ventilator during the day and sit down with her family to enjoy dinner. Suspensor straps were attached to the grid and backboard so that she could sit on a bicycle while still receiving ventilator support. She was able to improve her stamina and strength over a number of weeks, enabling her to get off the ventilator and join her family for a meal. With ventilator support, patients are capable of more work and more training, leaving them with better trained musculature. When they are off the ventilator, they are able to get through daily activities with less shortness of breath and better quality of life.

Techniques focusing on connective tissue release, muscle energy, and strain/counterstrain are remarkably effective in improving mobility and distance walked, even before beginning an endurance training program (Basmajian and Nyberg 1993). Mr. K. was a 60-year-old male with COPD and tuberculosis. In 1978, his vital capacity was 38%, expiratory flow rate 13%, and his PaO_2 was 69%. By 1981, his oxygen dropped to 52 at rest and 42 with exercise. He was started on oxygen, with some improvement in his PaO_2. Negative pressure nocturnal support was begun in 1983, when his PaO_2 dropped to 44%, his maximum volume ventilation (MVV) was 27%, his pimax was 34%, and his pemax was 10%. With nocturnal ventilator support, he showed rapid improvement: PaO_2 increased to 66%, pimax to 57%, and pemax to 43%. There were no changes in his breathing capacity. Rehabilitation began in 1986. In addition to severe restriction and limitation in thoracic, scapular, cervical, and lumbar mobility, he had remarkable anxiety about going outside and experiencing shortness of breath. With difficulty, he began walking, starting with a distance of 10 feet. Over the course of 2 years, he was walking 1 mile outdoors with low-flow oxygen. There was also a reversal from right-sided heart failure in 1986 with a left ventricular ejection fraction (LVEF) of 50% to an LVEF of 73% in 1988. The nocturnal support offered rest to the fatigued respiratory muscles and created the possibility for rehabilitation through improved mobility and ease of movement, as well as strength and endurance training.

The dynamics of breathing follow a pressure gradient that persists between the thoracic cavity and the abdominal cavity. As the negative pressure of the thorax increases, the positive pressure of the abdomen increases. One cavity relies on the pressure changes of the other; any change or restriction in one cavity will affect the function and efficiency of the other. An abdominal incision can cause increased abdominal pressure that can limit optimal thoracic expansion. Dr. B. was an 83-year-old male with a history of hypertension, hypercholesterolemia, arteriosclerotic heart disease, aortic insufficiency, coronary artery disease, and COPD (FEV_1 was 46% and MVV was 25% of predicted), who underwent open-heart surgery for a triple coronary bypass and aortic valve replacement in 1998. His postoperative course was complicated by difficulty in weaning off of the ventilator. He was sent home on bi-pap nocturnal support. His resting SaO_2 while on oxygen was 96 to 97. Evaluation showed markedly restricted thoracic expansion and a "bound down" sternum at the site of the surgical incision. Three sessions directed at releasing scar tissue and expanding thoracic and sterna mobility resulted in a resting SaO_2 of 97 off of oxygen. The saturation remained in the upper 90s with exercise, and subsequent sleep studies revealed that he no longer needed nocturnal ventilator support. The use of nocturnal support provided sufficient relief to allow therapeutic interventions that ultimately ended the patient's need for nocturnal support.

Summary

Nocturnal ventilator support is prescribed by a pulmonary specialist when patients with COPD show signs of increasing levels of $PaCO_2$, respiratory muscle fatigue, and/or sleep disorders. Although the criteria for use of nocturnal ventilator support are signs of progressing disease, the use of the ventilator can actually be a vehicle toward marked improvement. Patients and health providers often view the ventilator as a step closer to death, when in reality it can be a ticket to improved health and well-being. With the added breathing support that nocturnal ventilators provide, patients can be trained to improve breathing awareness and control, assume body positions that allow for better alignment, and be better able to tolerate therapeutic interventions aimed at improved mobility and flexibility. Ventilators can also be used to allow patients to undergo endurance training efforts that they would otherwise be incapable of performing. Manual therapies need to be an integral part of pulmonary rehabilitation. Clinical studies could easily be introduced to further evaluate the use of ventilators in rehabilitation of patients with COPD.

References

American Association for Respiratory Care. 1997. Consensus statement on non-invasive positive pressure ventilation. *Respir Care.* 42:362-369.

Basmajian, JV and R Nyberg. 1993. *Rational Manual Therapies.* Baltimore, MD: Williams & Wilkins.

Benditt, JO et al. 1997. Changes in breathing and ventilatory muscle recruitment patterns induced by lung volume reduction surgery. *Am J Respir Crit Care Med.* 155(1):279-284.

Berry, MJ. 1996. Inspiratory muscle training and whole body reconditioning in chronic obstructive pulmonary disease. *Am J Respir Crit Care Med.* 153:1812-1816.

Braun, NM and WD Marino. 1984. Effect of daily intermittent rest of respiratory muscles in patients with severe chronic airflow limitation. *Chest.* 85:59S-60S.

Breslin, EH. 1996. Respiratory muscle function in patients with COPD. *Heart & Lung.* 25(4):271-285.

Clini, E. 1998. Outcome of COPD patients performing nocturnal non-invasive mechanical ventilation. *Respir Med.* 929(10):1215-1222.

DeBruin et al. 1997. Size and strength of respiratory and quadraceps muscle in patients with chronic asthma. *Eur Respir J.* 10(1):59-64.

DeCramer, M. 1997. Hyperinflation and respiratory muscle interaction. *Eur Respir J.* 10(4):934-941.

DeTroyer et al. 1997. Neural drive to the diaphragm in patient with severe COPD. *Am J Respir Crit Care Med.* 155(4):1335-40.

DeTroyer et al. 1997. Effects of hyperinflation on the diaphragm. *Eur Respir J.* 10(3):708-713.

Dudley, DL, C Wermoth, and W Hague. 1973. Psychosocial aspects of care in the COPD patient. *Heart and Lung.* 2(3):389-393.

Ferrari, K. 1997. Chronic exertional dyspnea and respiratory muscle function in patients with COPD. *Lung.* 175(5):311-319.

Ferrari, K et al. 1997. Breathlessness and control of breathing in patients with COPD. *Monaldi Arch for Chest Dis.* 52(1):18-23.

Frownfelter, D and M Massery. 1996. Facilitating ventilation patterns and breathing strategies. In *Principals and Practice of Cardiopulmonary Physical Therapy*, D Frownfelter and E Dean. St. Louis, MO: Mosby.

Fujimoto, K et al. 1996. Effects of muscle relaxation therapy using specifically designed plates in patients with pulmonary emphysema. *Int Med.* 35(10):756-763.

Fujimoto, K. 1999. Improvement in thoracic movement following lung volume reduction surgery in patients with severe emphysema. *Int Med.* 38(2):119-125.

Georgopoulos, D et al. 1996. Control of breathing in mechanically ventilated patients. *Eur Respir J.* 9(10):2151-2160.

Gorini, M et al. 1996. Breathing pattern and carbon dioxide retention in severe COPD. *Thorax.* 51(7):677-683.

Heijdra, YF et al. 1996. Nocturnal saturation improves by target-flow inspiratory muscle training in patient with COPD. *Am J Respir Crit Care Med.* 153(1):260-265.

Ito, M et al. 1999. Immediate effects of respiratory muscle stretch gymnastics and diaphragmatic breathing in respiratory pattern. *Int Med.* 38(2):126-132.

Knuttgen, HG. 1979. Physical conditioning and limits to performance. In *Sports Medicine and Physiology*, RH Strauss. Philadelphia, PA: WB Saunders Co.

Kyroussis, D et al. 1996. Exhaustive exercise slows inspiratory muscle relaxation rate in chronic obstructive pulmonary disease. *Am J Respir Crit Care Med.* 153(2):787-793.

Miller, W. 1971. Useful methods of therapy. *Chest.* (Suppl.) 60:W2S-5S.

Nava, S. 1997. Patient-ventilator interaction and inspiratory effort during pressure support ventilation in patients with different pathologies. *Eur Respir J.* 10(1):177-183.

Rochester, DF, NMT Braun, and NS Arora. 1979. Respiratory muscle strength in chronic obstructive pulmonary disease. *Am Rev Respir Dis.* 119:151-154.

Saudny-Unterberger, H et al. 1997. Impact of nutritional support on functional status during an acute exacerbation of chronic obstructive pulmonary disease. *Am J Respir Crit Care Med.* 156:794-799.

Sliwinski, P. 1997. Inspiratory muscle dysfunction as a cause of death in COPD patients. *Monaldi Arch for Chest Dis.* 52(4):380-383.

Viale, JP. 1998. Time course evolution of ventilatory responses to inspiratory unloading in patients. *Am J Respir Crit Care Med.* 157(2):428-434.

3

Noninvasive Positive Pressure Ventilation With COPD/Emphysema

Debra Lierl, MEd, RRT, and Mike Chaney, RRT

Definition

Noninvasive positive pressure ventilation (NPPV) is the use of positive pressure ventilation without an invasive artificial airway. Nocturnal bilevel ventilation is the use of this two-pressure ventilation at night for a minimum of 4 hours per day. Ventilation is interfaced with the patient through a variety of available "masks" (nasal mask, full-face mask, or nasal pillows) that fit over the patient's mouth and nose or nose only. Positive pressure assists the patient during inhalation; exhalation is passive due to lung recoil. Diaphragmatic work can be eliminated if the inspiratory pressure is sufficient (Carrey et al 1984). Additionally, the majority of machines used for NPPV include positive end expiratory pressure (PEEP), which can be used to increase oxygenation and overcome the effects of auto-PEEP in patients with severe hyperinflation COPD (Appendini et al 1994). The term "bilevel ventilation" comes from the use of positive pressure support during inspiration (inspiratory positive airway pressure) to decrease the diaphragmatic work, decrease hypoventilation, and improve alveolar ventilation and the use of PEEP to improve oxygenation or decrease desaturation during sleep.

Physiology

Our lungs have 2 basic functions: one is to bring oxygen (O_2) to our bloodstream and the other is to remove carbon dioxide from our bodies. To do these tasks effectively, we must have sufficient respiratory drive, sufficient diaphragm and accessory muscle function and strength, and good lung function, including volumes and capacities to allow normal tidal breathing with enough reserve for increases in ventilatory workload when needed. During normal sleep, our PaO_2 drops slightly and our $PaCO_2$ rises slightly, secondary to shallow breathing. In the absence of lung disease, our bodies tolerate this fluctuation of decreased PaO_2 and increased $PaCO_2$ nicely. Our sleep is still deep enough and our rest is sufficient so that normal PaO_2 and $PaCO_2$ levels are restored upon waking with no side effects.

There are, however, certain diseases or conditions in which the decrease in PaO_2 and increase in $PaCO_2$ are exaggerated during sleep and not tolerated. Examples of these diseases include obstructive disorders such as COPD (emphysema, chronic bronchitis, bronchiectasis, cystic fibrosis), disorders of ventilatory control, neuromuscular disorders such as muscular dystrophy, and obesity hypoventilation syndrome. In all of these examples, lung function is compromised and, in severe cases, any fluctuation in PaO_2 or $PaCO_2$ or an increase in ventilatory workload is not tolerated because the patient is already at maximum workload just to maintain normal daytime tidal breathing. If during sleep these patients further desaturate or hypoventilate, the side effect is compromised daytime lung function and decreased ability to perform activities of daily living.

Theory and Studies

Hyperinflation in patients with COPD increases the work of breathing (Hill et al 1999). Due to the increased work of breathing with hyperinflation in the COPD patient, it was first suggested that there may be some benefit to resting the patient's chronically fatigued muscles by the use of NPPV nocturnally (Braun et al 1984, Nava et al 1993, Rentson et al 1994). It was further theorized that this period of rest (4 to 6 hours per day) would permit recovery of muscle, increase muscle strength, reduce the periods of muscle fatigue, and improve gas exchange as well as pulmonary function values (Hill et al). Some studies have shown improvement of the respiratory muscles with the use of NPPV (Braun et al, Cropp and DiMarco 1987, Gutierrez et al 1988, Scano et al 1990, Ambrosino et al 1990), while other studies found no benefit in the use of NPPV (Zibrak et al 1988, Celli et al 1989, Shapiro et al 1992). The studies that found improvement also correlated the improvement to the reduction of the $PaCO_2$ rather than the improvement of the respiratory muscle strength (Juan et al 1984, Hill et al). Hill also points out that the favorable studies showed an average baseline $PaCO_2$ 10 mm Hg greater than the unfavorable studies. This fact stresses how important patient selection is for successful use of nocturnal NPPV.

Nocturnal Complications

The following are side effects of people with lung disease who are not tolerating the changes in PaO_2 and $PaCO_2$ during sleep and who may have exaggerated changes (nocturnal hypoventilation). These may be used to assess a patient for NPPV therapy.

- Daytime sleepiness and frequent napping due to the body's not going into a deep enough sleep to allow sufficient rest.
- Increased daytime $PaCO_2$ levels secondary to insufficient diaphragmatic rest during sleep. Another theory is that the possible large fluctuation in

$PaCO_2$ may actually contribute to raising the central chemoreceptor sensitivity to a higher CO_2 level (lower pH level).

- Morning headaches due to increased $PaCO_2$ and decreased PaO_2 levels. These headaches usually go away after the patient has been up for a while.
- Poor sleep with frequent awakening, probably due to hypoxemic episodes and shallow sleep.
- Poor appetite.
- Poor memory and concentration from insufficient rest.
- Fatigue that comes easily due to insufficient rest.
- Frequent hospitalizations (Smith 1998). Poor sleep does not allow for adequate muscular rest required to have the strength to generate an adequate cough. The immune system can also be compromised if the patient is run down due to poor sleep.
- Exacerbations or development of cor pulmonale secondary to chronic hypoxemic pulmonary vasoconstriction evidenced by orthopnea (patient will sleep with multiple pillows and/or may exhibit pedal edema).
- Increased work of breathing during the day.
- O_2 desaturations at night from shallow breathing, obstructive components of the upper airway, poor distribution of ventilation (shunted areas from atelectasis, mucous), or hypoventilation (increased $PaCO_2$ levels).

How NPPV Works

Patients with severe COPD are known to have a high incidence of sleep-disordered breathing, including sleep apnea, and periods of hypoventilation with oxygen desaturation (Fleetham et al 1982). They are also known to have poor quality of sleep and shorter sleep times (Catterall et al 1983). Since continuous positive airway pressure (CPAP) and bilevel positive airway pressure have been shown to improve sleep in the non-COPD, it was theorized that they would also help the COPD patients. Sleep studies have shown an improvement of sleep in COPD patients using NPPV. The two pressures used during NPPV are usually referred to as inspiratory positive airway pressure (IPAP) and expiratory positive airway pressure (EPAP). EPAP is a constant minimum set pressure delivered to the airway, which has the same function as PEEP or CPAP. It can splint the airway open to offset upper airway obstructions and help prevent premature airway collapse. It can improve compliance and distribution of ventilation and collateral ventilation and will also increase mean airway pressure. This can normalize PaO_2 levels at night, thereby improving the conditions and side effects that go with it. When the patient inhales, the NPPV machine will increase to a higher set pressure, the IPAP. This change to a higher pressure will increase the patient's tidal volume, which improves or can normalize $PaCO_2$ levels. IPAP has the same function as pressure support ventilation.

The IPAP portion of this therapy can also take some of the workload imposed on the diaphragm, allowing it to rest during sleep. Through improving PaO_2 and $PaCO_2$ and decreasing the workload of breathing during sleep, we improve cardiovascular function, decrease daytime sleepiness, work of breathing and fatigue, rid the patient of morning headaches, reduce hospitalizations, and improve muscular strength, which can improve cough and reserve volumes. By improving strength and reserve volumes, the patient's level of activity is improved. By stabilizing the $PaCO_2$ levels to a relatively normal level at night, the central chemoreceptors can theoretically not only be kept from rising but may actually reset to a lower level. Appetite, memory, and concentration may also improve from sufficient rest, which can happen because of the patient's going into a deeper sleep.

Quotes From Patients

Although the studies supporting NPPV are not conclusive, patients who have benefited from its use are very strong in their endorsement. Jonathan Waugh from Georgia State University is currently working on a study titled "The Effect of Noninvasive Positive Pressure Ventilation on Patients with Chronic Hypercapnia." His study is investigating quality of life issues as well as hospital admissions. Although this study has not been completed, a preliminary report documents patients' perception of their improvement:

"I can walk further and play basketball and swim. I operate a nonprofit radio station in my home."

"I can sleep a lot better; I can get my breath better; I can walk to the mailbox and back and couldn't before. I can walk around the house."

"I can sleep better, don't cough as much."

"Can walk a lot further, can do mild exercise, take showers, drive, prepare food for meals."

Consensus Conference Recommendation

A national consensus conference was organized and convened by the National Association for Medical Direction of Respiratory Care in Washington, DC, in 1998. The report from this conference, published in the August 1999 issue of *Chest*, reported that although there seems to be a need for more controlled long-term studies, NPPV ventilation seems to be better tolerated than negative pressure ventilation in the COPD patient. The report also documented improvement for COPD patients with obstructive sleep apnea (Hill et al 1999). Patients with little or no CO_2 retention do not seem to benefit from NPPV, whereas patients with CO_2 retention above 50 mm Hg do. If the patient additionally exhibits desaturation during sleep, the benefit from NPPV is even greater (Hill et al).

Clinical Indicators as Agreed to by Consensus Conference Participants
(*Chest*, August 1999, p. 529)

1. Disease documentation
   i. Before considering a COPD patient for NPPV, a physician with skills and experience in NPPV must establish and document an appropriate diagnosis on the basis of history, physical examination, and results of diagnostic tests and assure optimal management of COPD with such treatments as bronchodilators, oxygen when indicated, and optimal management of other underlying disorders (such as performing a multichannel sleep study to exclude associated sleep apnea if clinically indicated).
   ii. The most common obstructive lung diseases would include chronic bronchitis, emphysema, bronchiectasis, and cystic fibrosis.
2. Indications for usage
   i. Symptoms (such as fatigue, dyspnea, morning headache, etc) and
   ii. Physiologic criteria (one of the following)
      a. $PaCO_2 > 55$ mm Hg
      b. $PaCO_2$ of 50 to 54 mm Hg and nocturnal desaturation (oxygen saturation by pulse oximeter $< 88\%$ for 5 continuous minutes while receiving oxygen therapy $2 > L/$ min)
      c. $PaCO_2$ of 50 to 54 mm Hg and hospitalization related to recurrent (> 2 in a 12-month period) episodes of hypercapnic respiratory failure

Setting Pressures

"[NPPV] must be administered through a trained clinician because the patient will go through a period in which he or she will have to adapt to it. There will be many hurdles encountered along the way during that period, and the clinician needs to know how to help the patient overcome them." (Smith 1998, p. 92). In fact, when reviewing most of the studies, the reason for poor results or small numbers of participants is due to poor patient compliance. As a starting point, an IPAP pressure of 8 mm Hg and an EPAP pressure of 4 mm Hg is generally used. Protocols should be used for adjusting the pressure. IPAP should be increased to improve alveolar ventilation or the $PaCO_2$ and the EPAP should be increased to improve oxygenation and/or obstructed sleep apnea. It is important to remember that if the EPAP is increased, the practitioner must also increase the IPAP to maintain the same pressure difference. The minimum EPAP level is recommended as 4 mm Hg by most manufacturers. If oxygen is needed, it can be bled in. Most manufacturers publish a bleed-in chart for oxygen to help the practitioner maintain the patient's ordered liter flow or percentage.

Monitoring

Patients should be monitored on a regular basis. Monitoring should include the parameters that were used for patient selection. Additionally, patients should be monitored for symptomatic relief, increased level of daytime activity, signs of cor pulmonale or pedal edema, and respiratory rate. In most cases, the practitioner should see an improvement in the patient's resting respiratory rate, oxygen saturation, increased level of activity, decreased $PaCO_2$, and fewer hospital admissions.

How This Fits Into Palliative Care

All medical therapy for the COPD patient may yield only marginal benefits, but even small improvements may lead to significant functional benefits, improving the quality of life. Due to the life expectancy of the patient with severe COPD, it may be difficult to conduct long-term studies with a large population. For the correctly selected patient who is compliant and willing to accept this form of therapy, the results have been significant in improving activities of daily living function and improving quality of life.

References

Ambrosino, N, T Montagna, S Nava et al. 1990. Short term effect of intermittent negative pressure ventilation in COPD patients with respiratory failure. *Eur Respir J.* 3:502-508.

Ambrosino, N, S Nava, P Bertone, C Fracchia, and C Rampulla. 1992. Physiologic evaluation of pressure support ventilation by nasal mask in patients with stable COPD. *Chest.* 101:385-391.

Appendini, L, A Palessio, S Zanaboni et al. 1994. Physiologic effects of positive end expiratory pressure and mask pressure support during exacerbations of chronic obstructive pulmonary disease. *Am J Respir Crit Care Med.* 149:1069-1076.

Braun, NM and WD Marino. 1984. Effect of daily intermittent rest of respiratory muscles in patients with severe chronic airflow limitation. *Chest.* 85:59S-60S.

Carrey, Z, SB Gottfried, and RD Levy. 1984. Ventilatory muscle support in respiratory failure with nasal positive pressure ventilation. *Chest.* 97:150-158.

Catterall, JR, NJ Douglas, PMA Calverley et al. 1983. Transient hypoxemia during sleep in chronic obstructive pulmonary disease is not a sleep apnea syndrome. *Am Rev Respir Dis.* 128:24-29.

Celli, B, H Lee, C Criner et al. 1989. Controlled trial of external negative pressure ventilation in patients with severe airflow obstruction. *Am Rev Respir Dis.* 140:1251-1256.

Cropp, A and A DiMarco. 1987. Effects of intermittent negative pressure ventilation on respiratory muscle function in patients with severe chronic obstructive pulmonary disease. *Am Rev Respir Dis.* 135:1056-1061.

Fleetham, J, P West, B Mezon et al. 1982. Sleep, aerosol and oxygen desaturation in chronic obstructive pulmonary disease. *Am Rev Respir Dis.* 126:429-433.

Gutierrez, M, T Berolza, G Contreras et al. 1988. Weekly cuirass ventilation improves blood gases and inspiratory muscle strength in patients with chronic airflow limitation and hypercarbia. *Am Rev Respir Dis.* 138:617-623.

Hill, N, P Leger, and G Criner. 1999. Clinical indications for noninvasive positive pressure ventilation in chronic respiratory failure due to restrictive lung disease, COPD, and nocturnal hypoventilation: a consensus conference report. *Chest.* 116:521-534.

Juan, G, P Calverley, C Talamo et al. 1984. Effect of carbon dioxide on diaphragmatic function in human beings. *N Engl J Med.* 310:874-879.

Nava, S, N Ambrosino, F Rubini et al. 1993. Effect of nasal pressure support ventilation and external PEEP on diaphragmatic activity in patients with severe stable COPD. *Chest.* 103:143-150.

Renston, JP, AF DiMarco, and GS Supinski. 1994. Respiratory muscle rest using nasal biPAP ventilation in patients with stable severe COPD. *Chest.* 105:1053-1060.

Scano, C, F Gigliotti, R Duranti et al. 1990. Changes in ventilatory muscle function with negative pressure ventilation in patients with severe COPD. *Chest.* 97:322-332.

Shapiro, SH, P Ernst, K Gray-Donald et al. 1992. Effect of negative pressure ventilation in severe chronic obstructive pulmonary disease. *Lancet.* 340:1425-1429.

Smith, R. 1998. Noninvasive mechanical ventilation. *Home Health Care Dealer/ Supplier.* Nov-Dec: 91-93.

Zibrak, JD, NS Hill, ED Federman et al. 1988. Evaluation of intermittent long-term negative pressure ventilation in patients with severe chronic obstructive pulmonary disease. *Am Rev Respir Dis.* 138:1515-1518.

4

Thriving, Not Just Surviving:
Practical Techniques for Living With
Mechanical Ventilation

Barbara Rogers

The author is director of Breethezy™*, an education, recovery, and support program developed to address the needs of the ventilator community in the emerging technologically oriented home care market. Breethezy is a multidimensional program derived from a patient's experience in transition from ventilator resistance to full acceptance, and also draws from traditional and innovative recovery and rehabilitation programs, including the 12-step modality.*

Changes in the American health care system are resulting in fewer hospitalizations, shorter stays, and a market-based approach to health care financing—patients are being sent home sooner but sometimes are still sick. New procedures are saving lives, but are leaving many patients with long-term care needs. Today, chronic illnesses rather than acute illnesses are the most prevalent forms of disease, and advanced technology has moved from hospitals to homes as well. We now have the ability to treat many patients with chronic illnesses at home in a way that is more economical than hospitalization and that offers a better quality of life. However, this rapidly advancing technology often leaves many health care professionals who are unfamiliar with the equipment provided treating ventilator users in the home setting. Also, because of changing reimbursement schedules, family caregivers are an essential part of today's evolving health care network. They are expected to take on more responsibility for longer periods with less support. Current home care protocol must include examining the new and expanded needs of ventilator users, families, caregivers, and health care professionals; these participants must be provided initial and ongoing education, training, and emotional support.

Health care in the United States is a trillion dollar enterprise. Research by the United Hospital Fund (Arno and Levine 1998) estimated that the median cost in 1996 of replacing family caregiving with professional care was $194 billion—19% of total health care expenditures. In 1994, the annual cost of care for a ventilator-dependent person in a hospital was

$271,000. Comparable care at home cost less than $22,000. That is a saving of $249,000, or a 92% reduction in cost. This disparity increases annually. Home care is one of the few ways in which cost-conscious insurers can simultaneously save money and increase patient satisfaction. Patients at home recover faster and live longer than those in institutions, and home care helps keep families intact and gives the ill and disabled a greater degree of comfort and dignity. Technical advances and economic advantages are making it more possible to return health care to the home, where it began centuries ago. This is where patients find the greatest satisfaction and quality of life.

The number and types of ventilators in the home care market continue to expand so rapidly that communication breaks down between medical device manufacturers, distributors, and users. Unless they have had special, ongoing training, owners and staff of small firms, and even home health agency nurses, may be unfamiliar with new home ventilators. Also, in many locations throughout the United States, ventilator patients do not have access to specialists and are treated by their primary care physicians. These physicians are often not very familiar with the equipment they are prescribing, and even those who are, including specialists, often have little training or experience in the home care setting. Of the 123 US medical schools, only one third require students to have a home care experience. In some programs, this experience consists of a single home visit. Only 3 US medical schools require all students to make 6 or more home visits in their clinical years.

People dependent on ventilators are coming home in unprecedented numbers. When treating these ventilator users in their homes, health care professionals have to go beyond the treatment of the disease itself. Additional factors impact recovery. Therefore, the transition of the ventilator user to the home setting must be a process rather than a single event, requiring a team effort focusing on organization, communication, and support. There is a proven gap between having the equipment and tools for recovery and using them successfully. The tools that can help many patients, and in some cases save lives, are often the very tools that can produce fear and anxiety, preventing them from being used as prescribed.

A primary cause of fear is loss of control, which increases a feeling of vulnerability and makes it difficult for ventilator users to feel safe in their environment. This is especially true when dealing with something as basic as breathing and when patients are homebound, often not able to use mobility to help themselves. When ventilator users take back some control by participating in their recovery, they feel safer and more empowered. Understanding of and participation in the process of recovery have a positive effect on attitude and help eliminate a victim mentality that impedes compliance and recovery. The same applies to families and caregivers who are often as traumatized as, or more traumatized than, the ventilator users themselves by the ventilator users' state. In addition, patients are often unable to make the cause-and-effect connection between certain issues and how they inhibit recovery, issues that only communication and teamwork will reveal.

Breethezy Methods

Breethezy employs a team care concept combined with seminars and workshops, hands-on experiential education for health care professionals, and networks of support systems and "tools" for ventilator users, their families, and caregivers. This approach produces a more successful compliance and recovery outcome than these efforts would individually. The Breethezy team care concept is similar to that of an orchestra, with the patient being the composition and the physician being the conductor. The program strives to have all the players in the orchestra working together, or harmonizing, to create a smooth flowing experience.

The team consists of patient and family support systems, physicians, respiratory therapists, and other health care professionals, all interacting and working together. The results are better service for patients, a safe living experience, expanded functional living, and increased compliance. The mental, physical, and emotional health of patients are the primary concerns, and care is customized to fit their specific needs, thereby increasing positive outcomes.

Breethezy addresses 3 main components to successful compliance: quality of life, transition to home, and clinical applications (matching the machine to the patient).

Quality of Life

Frequently, patients facing the use of a ventilator for the first time are not in good mental or physical condition. They are often fearful of the prospect of mechanical ventilation and of the very equipment itself, and denial may be an additional factor. It is hard for many patients to understand why they now need this therapy and how they arrived at this state. For COPD patients, where no specific "trauma" such as an accident or fall occurred to which they can link this turn of events, it is often more difficult to arrive at acceptance and compliance than it is for other ventilator users. Patients with chronic and degenerative diseases that have progressed over a period of years have an especially difficult time accepting the need for mechanical intervention. By the time the need for a ventilator arrives, these patients are frequently depressed and despondent, with a sense of hopelessness. High CO_2 build-up and low O_2 saturation are often contributory factors, and can also produce irritability and personality changes.

In addition, patients fear loss of function. They anticipate a loss of independence and are fearful of being a burden on their families and loved ones. In addition, many patients face their own mortality for the first time, with

29

the thought of not seeing loved ones taken care of or children and grandchildren grown becoming more of a reality.

Patients also grapple with loss of image and socialization in our very image-conscious and social culture. Isolation, difficulty traveling, and logistical problems all become issues to deal with. As a result, patients often feel alone, with no one to identify with, no peers with whom to discuss and communicate these concerns.

Ventilator users need to realize that they can indeed have quality of life while using mechanical ventilation. It is also important for them to participate in their own care and recovery. Participation is empowering and helps to eliminate or reduce the fear brought on by loss of control. Breethezy addresses these areas by creating networks and support systems through which patients and families can meet and communicate with others in similar situations. So much is gained by exchanging information with others traveling the same road, because no one can speak on a subject as well as someone who has been there and done that. It is a valuable opportunity to see the "light at the end of the tunnel" from others' successes, and to be able to provide that light to those just starting out on the road or perhaps stalled along the way. Discussing experiences, problems, solutions, and "life" with someone who can relate first-hand is invaluable; it lifts one's spirits in a way that nothing else can and encourages participation in one's own care and recovery. Patients are also encouraged to talk about their problems, fears, and concerns and to tell their stories, as this too is very freeing.

Breethezy uses similar networks for professional interaction within the ventilator community. With the world changing so quickly, professionals need to be able to exchange ideas with others who have found creative solutions to similar situations. Breethezy also encourages the patient/family community and the professional community to interact with each other to provide a better understanding of each group's specific experiences.

Transition to Home

Breathing is so basic a need that anything that affects it often produces fear and anxiety. When a patient is ready to transition to the home setting, there is frequently a fear of not being able to replicate the safe environment of the hospital or health care facility. A patient tends to focus on the possibility of machine malfunctions or power failures. Household logistics loom large on the horizon and, with them, fear of the physical and financial burdens of caregiving on the patient's family. Equally threatening is the reduction of dignity that often comes with the family assuming responsibility for the most personal of physical needs and bodily functions.

Patients may also fear improvement and self-responsibility. If they were to regain some independence, some patients fear that they will lose their skilled caregivers and "guards." This concern is often disturbing enough to prevent patients from achieving their best recovery and living the fullest possible life. All the factors that go into successful adaptation and compliance must be recognized so that a safe and acceptable plan of care can be designed. Patients should not see improvement as resulting in a reduction of the support systems that they rely on, a positive action producing a negative result. One female patient rejected therapy and kept herself in an invalid state because she feared losing her full-time nurses and being alone if she regained any self-reliance. To ease her transition back to self-care and independence, Breethezy worked with the patient and family and offered to replace her nurses with a nonskilled companion as she recovered.

Family members are often even more traumatized than the ventilator user as they deal with many of the same issues. In addition, they are frequently faced with the added responsibility of participating in the care and upkeep of the new equipment. The family's issues and needs must be recognized and addressed, as well as those of the patient. It is also important to offer family members an outlet, separate from the patient's, through which to identify and discuss their needs and feelings.

Clinical Applications: Matching the Machine to the Patient

There are many methods of mechanical ventilation available and numerous ventilators, each having its own personal characteristics. Of utmost importance when choosing the correct mode for a patient is compatibility to that patient. When setting up a patient with a ventilator, his or her own breathing should be replicated as closely as possible. For example, the patient's natural number of breaths per minute should be observed and the ventilator should be set to that number at the start. Too many times patients have complained that the ventilator "breathes against them" and they cannot use it. Just because a patient's oxygen saturation or other numbers are in line does not mean that the set-up is correct. Numbers are not enough. A set-up must be comfortable to the patient, as well as clinically acceptable, to achieve a positive outcome.

Health care professionals need to be creative. They should try various types of machines and modes of delivery. Selecting the appropriate ventilator and interface for a patient is like buying a pair of shoes—a person must try them on and wear them a bit to see if the shoes fit comfortably. It is very important to match the machine to the patient. Often by keeping an open mind and reconfiguring equipment—not necessarily in textbook format—health care professionals can find a more comfortable and clinically acceptable solution for a patient.

Of course, with today's reimbursement criteria, it is not fiscally feasible to present and allow patients to try every mask and interface that is on the market. However, health care professionals should let patients know about the various options that are available. Also, patients should be familiarized with the different fine-tuning adjustments during equipment set-up. Most patients have no idea of what goes into "creating" a breath. They do not break a breath down into its parts, such as force, inspiratory length, volume, pressure, or rate, nor are they aware of settings such as plateaus or sighs. It is important to clearly explain to patients what each of these terms means and how fine-tuning each control will affect the way the breath is delivered and feels. Otherwise, getting a ventilator set up is like going to buy a pair of shoes and not knowing that they come in different sizes and widths. In addition to educating patients, this interaction also includes patients in the selection process, creating a better acceptance of the final choice. Other factors to pay attention to are such things as claustrophobia, running or dry nose, and mouth breathing. These are issues that, while often easily remedied, can undermine successful compliance if not addressed.

"Missing Link" Issues

Included in Breethezy's clinical applications component is a subcomponent of nonclinical problems that prevent compliance. We call these the "missing link" issues. Patients and families cannot always understand why certain problems inhibit compliance. Therefore, looking at the "total" patient and his or her environment is often critical in determining and addressing these issues. Most failures are because of such missing link issues rather than to clinical/mechanical issues. Breethezy has developed several "recovery" tools to help patients and families address such issues. Health care professionals must work with ventilator users to become familiar with these tools and to encourage patients and their families to use them. Also, having a good understanding of a patient's day-to-day needs and concerns is necessary to fill in these missing links and help the patient achieve the best possible outcome.

Because isolation is one of the biggest problems that patients with respiratory illness face, ways must be provided to establish a support network and develop friendships. The exchange of information, hope, and insight and sometimes just the confirmation from a fellow patient that it is, in fact, "a crummy breathing day" are very important. This communication can be achieved over the telephone and via the Internet. Doctors and home care companies should introduce patients with similar situations to each other and develop local networks and resources. Interaction is a positive, empowering action. The chat room on the Breethezy Web site (www.breethezy.com) is an excellent source of interaction and resources for ventilator users and families, and is a wonderful tool for the transition period as well as for ongoing participation and recovery. The Internet is also a wonderful resource for available services and materials. Personal computers have opened up a new world of possibilities to those with physical limitations.

A personal journal also can prove very helpful. Often, patients do not think they are making progress at all, and it is easy for them to feel depressed and unmotivated. During these times, it is useful to be able to look back over the past few months and see the progress that has been made. Small steps are still steps and a small amount of progress is still progress, facts that need to be reinforced.

A Personal Commitment Sheet on which patients can plan activities and goals for the upcoming week (or day, or month, etc.) is another useful tool. Therapies, exercises, meditation—any activity that is important to the patient—should be included. Writing these activities down and thereby formally committing to them frequently proves productive. When doing this, realistic and attainable goal setting is crucial to a patient's emotional well-being and state of mind. Helping patients to establish goals that they can achieve, and thereby feel successful and good about themselves, is very important. Although it is good for patients to have long-term as well as short-term plans, goals that may be attainable in the future but that are not immediately achievable should be chosen carefully because patients can be left feeling defeated.

Along with the Personal Commitment Sheet, patients should use an Accomplishment Check-off Sheet on which they can mark off accomplishments and see physical evidence of achievement. Seeing this evidence of success in black and white reinforces forward strides. It is uplifting and validating and can become a source of pride in their commitment to themselves.

Program Results

- Customized care in setting up the ventilator—carefully tailoring it to patients' specific needs—results in better adaptation to and use of the equipment.

- When patients and their families participate in the process of choosing and adjusting the equipment, there appears to be a reduction in the anxiety and fear associated with using and maintaining it after the health care professional leaves.

- Patients who have a support system for nonclinical or "missing link" issues have better transition and better compliance to a prescribed plan of care than those patients without such support.

- The use of material and visual aids, such as commitment sheets, accomplishment sheets, and personal journals, keeps patients mentally active and "in the process." Such tangible evidence of effort and results helps to keep patients focused on positive activities and shows them that they indeed can have a "life." This is uplifting and validating, and helps to relieve depression.

- Although Breethezy has not done clinical trials, the group of patients worked with who have these support systems and customized care have reduced hospitalizations. These patients also tend to be more satisfied with their quality of life.

- Health care professionals who use Breethezy's "total patient" approach build a better rapport with their patients. These professionals also gain a greater and more intimate knowledge of the equipment they work with and the process that their patients experience.

Ventilator patients transition better and achieve a higher degree of compliance when a support system is available that customizes their clinical care as well as addresses their nonclinical issues and needs.

Resources

Arno, PS and C Levine. 1998. *Economic Value of Informal Caregiving in the United States*. Families and Health Care Project: United Hospital Fund.

Borfitz, D. 1988. Home is where the health care is. *FDA Consumer*. 22:34.

Fusco, R. 1994. Home care: an emerging solution to the healthcare crisis. *Hospital Topics*. 72:32.

5

South to Alaska:
Traveling With Mechanical Ventilation

Phil Petersen

Some of what seems surprising to academia today, even after a decade of research and data collecting, was known and well understood by my late wife and me back in the latter 1980s. We knew about pulmonary illness, allergies, respiratory rehabilitation, lack of muscle strength, mental and physical fatigue, emotions, and motivation. Yes, we knew a lot about chronic obstructive pulmonary disease (COPD).

While in the Canadian Arctic, my wife, Mary B., developed a bad infection, a nasty cold that she could not shake, which made breathing difficult. After stopping at a small village clinic and spending $25 on tests (including laboratory, breathing, and x-ray), she was told that she had COPD. Even though we were somewhat shocked, we still had to make up our minds as to what this illness would do to our future.

We were well aware she would soon be required to have supplemental oxygen and wondered if it would lead to becoming a shut-in, like a friend we knew on oxygen. Now, years later, I use a big word—reclusive—to describe what could have happened to her. Instead, we made up our minds to resist becoming reclusive. To do this, she would need stamina, and both of us would need to acquire as much practical knowledge about her illness as possible. Indeed, so many people with lung disease withdraw from the world because, lacking knowledge, the cards are stacked against them. "Knowledge" is another key word.

One year later, Mary B. came home from the hospital after 2 weeks in the intensive care unit. She was dragging a 21-pound "portable" oxygen E-tank behind her. Given her weakened condition, her doctor, even a decade ago, could have prescribed a truly portable unit. Instead, he simply had his nurse arrange with the oxygen company to "supply Mrs. Petersen with oxygen." Physicians still do this today, as many lack the information or the knowledge to do otherwise. How can they educate their patients, if they don't even bother to find out what happens to those patients on the way home, and after they get home? This is the point where reclusiveness sets in.

We started investigating. The home-care company that was supplying the oxygen was of very little help. It received the same fee for oxygen, no matter in what form it was dispensed. Mary B. had all the oxygen she required, including spare tanks, but it was the lack of truly modern equipment that hampered her quality of life. Fortunately, however, a nurse friend happened to see a new type of small portable oxygen unit at a medical equipment supplier. It was what we today call a "pulse-dose conserver" system for compressed gas. We purchased the unit with ten miniature oxygen tanks and maintained the equipment ourselves, including having the tanks filled at a welding supply company. The tanks were so small that a couple of extras could be carried in a shopping bag, allowing almost unlimited time away from home. As a result, Mary B. was truly mobile for the next few years.

Today, these portable conservers weigh five pounds and last as long as an E-tank, and the oxygen supplier rents them to patients at about the same cost as it would to an insurer. For the past few years, doctors have been able to prescribe either compressed or liquid oxygen and *if* portable oxygen is also prescribed, the home-care company must, to the best of my knowledge, supply a portable unit with adequate tanks for unrestricted mobility. If the patient arrives at the doctor's office dragging an E-tank, the physician should immediately take steps to correct the grave injustice.

Not only have doctors been slow to adapt to these changes, but the Health Care Financing Administration (HCFA) resists any change in setting guidelines for Medicare, even if it improves the quality of life of its constituency, often at a lower cost.

As Mary B.'s condition worsened, we found that a wheelchair was a necessity. It was sort of a lifeline at first, but it became a means of keeping Mary B. ambulatory. Because of lack of muscle strength, particularly in her arms, we really did not have much desire to manipulate one of those unwieldy standard wheelchairs with the big wheels weighing about 50 pounds. A travelchair with four small wheels (sometimes called a transportchair) was the answer. It weighed less than 20 pounds, was easy to store (even on airlines), and I could lift it out of my car's trunk without straining my back. The mobility prevented Mary B. from becoming reclusive.

Medicare? I don't know. A travelchair costs a little less money than a standard wheelchair and is more practical for those dependent on oxygen. In my opinion, however, Medicare would rather pay for the more expensive piece of equipment. HCFA needs to make some comparisons. Regardless, getting out of the house by whatever means possible involves exercise of the mind and body, combating that demon "reclusiveness." By not being reclusive, Mary B. had no visits to the emergency room and was able to visit her doctor on a regular basis—all in all, not running up big expenses for Medicare.

To professionals dealing with lung patients: I urge you to acquire the knowledge to enable you to prescribe proper equipment and stand up against insurers through your associations. Encourage those associations to be active in areas that affect the well-being of your patients. Talk to the home-care company staff, get to know their equipment, and then talk to their competitors.

My wife died 7 years ago on the way to her doctor's office. That trip didn't cost Medicare a penny.

6

Lung Transplantation for COPD

Larry L. Schulman, MD

In 1970, a report in the *New England Journal of Medicine* demonstrated that single lung transplantation for advanced pulmonary emphysema was technically possible, but raised serious questions whether the procedure was physiologically feasible (Stevens et al 1970). In two patients with advanced pulmonary emphysema, the authors observed hyperinflation of the native emphysematous lung associated with reduced volume and ventilation to the transplant lung. The authors concluded that "patients with emphysema may be poor candidates for lung transplantation" (Stevens et al). Eighteen years later, after successful single lung transplantation for pulmonary fibrosis (Toronto Lung Transplant Group 1988), thoracic surgeons revisited earlier attempts at lung transplantation for patients with pulmonary emphysema. We now understand that the two earliest single lung transplant recipients for pulmonary emphysema died because of diffuse pneumonitis in the transplant lung, and that gross ventilation and perfusion imbalances after single lung transplantation are not physiologically inevitable or insurmountable (Cooper 1997). Nevertheless, as will be discussed below, many of the issues raised in 1970 are still relevant, such as hyperinflation of the native lung and reduced volume and ventilation to the transplant lung.

Several excellent general reviews of lung transplantation have been published recently (Trulock 1997, Arcasoy and Kotloff 1999). The remainder of this paper will focus on lung transplantation for advanced pulmonary emphysema. The discussion will be divided into three broad categories:

1. Optimal candidate selection
2. Physiology of the transplanted lung
3. Risks and benefits of lung transplantation

Optimal Candidate Selection

An unexpected consequence of successful lung transplantation for pulmonary emphysema was a reevaluation of the clinician's approach and nomenclature for chronic airflow obstruction. The tendency to lump a variety of conditions under the rubric "chronic obstructive pulmonary disease" (COPD) was disadvantageous in selecting appropriate candidates for lung transplantation. The ideal candidate for lung transplantation recalled the original description of patients with emphysema (Type A COPD), namely, those patients with little cough, occasional and scanty sputum, fixed dyspnea, thin body habitus, large translucent lungs with low diaphragms and small cardiothoracic ratio, absence of right ventricular enlargement, and a normal hematocrit (Nash et al 1965). Optimal candidates for lung transplantation should not manifest reversible airflow obstruction, copious sputum production, respiratory infection, obesity, or respiratory muscle weakness. By these criteria, optimal candidates tend to manifest less severe derangements of gas exchange (hypoxemia and hypercarbia) and less severe elevations of pulmonary arterial pressures (Schulman et al 1994).

The criteria may be relaxed for patients who are being considered for bilateral lung transplantation, especially regarding sputum production and respiratory infection. Sputum production and respiratory infection may be eradicated by the transplant surgery, similar to bilateral lung transplantation for patients with idiopathic bronchiectasis or cystic fibrosis. By the expanded criteria, candidates for bilateral lung transplantation may manifest more severe derangements of gas exchange and elevation of pulmonary arterial pressures.

Patients should be referred for transplantation when FEV_1 % predicted falls below 25% to 30% (Joint Statement ... American Thoracic Society 1988). For patients with alpha 1-antitrypsin deficiency, survival data have been well-defined, reflecting the fact that these are younger patients with a more "pure" form of pulmonary emphysema. The Alpha 1-Antitrypsin Deficiency Registry Study Group detected a 30% 5-year mortality rate for patients with FEV_1 % predicted at less than 35%, which was only insignificantly better for patients who were receiving enzyme replacement therapy (Alpha 1-Antitrypsin Deficiency Registry Study Group 1995). For patients with pulmonary emphysema unrelated to alpha 1-antitrypsin deficiency, survival data are more variable, reflecting greater heterogeneity of age and disease. In the IPPB trial, 3-year mortality was 33% for patients whose FEV_1 % predicted was less than 30% and who were below 60 years of age, but 55% for patients 60 years and older (Anthonisen 1989). For patients with FEV_1 % predicted at 30% to 39%, 3-year mortality was 15% for patients below 60 years of age, and 35% for patients 60 years and older. For patients with disturbances in gas exchange, elevated $PaCO_2$ associated with acute exacerbations were strong predictors of mortality (Gray-Donald et al 1996).

Patients with advanced pulmonary emphysema should meet general guidelines for lung transplant candidates. The general criteria have been published recently as an international consensus statement (Joint Statement ... American Thoracic Society 1988). The discussion in this chapter will focus on criteria specific for patients with advanced pulmonary emphysema.

Optimal candidates for single lung transplantation should be 65 years of age or younger; for bilateral lung transplantation, 60 years of age or younger. All candidates must be ambulatory (one study has indicated that a 6-minute walk distance less than 300 m is predictive of poor outcome) and must participate in a supervised pulmonary rehabilitation program. Patients' weight should not be below 70% of ideal body weight, nor exceed 130% of ideal body weight. Candidates should have adequate social support and prescription medication coverage and should demonstrate motivation, with a willingness and an ability to adhere to an intensive medical regimen after surgery. Global assessment of psychosocial "risk" before transplantation has been predictive of noncompliance with medication regimen, diet, exercise, and smoking abstinence after transplantation.

Candidates for lung transplantation should not have coronary artery disease or left ventricular dysfunction (since many candidates are former smokers, transplant centers frequently require preoperative coronary arteriography), nor should they be acutely or critically ill at the time of the transplant. Mechanically ventilated patients have been demonstrated to have poor postoperative outcomes related to infection and respiratory muscle weakness. Ambulatory patients who have a chronic tracheostomy for nocturnal ventilation may be eligible for transplantation. Non-invasive mechanical ventilation, such as BIPAP mask, is acceptable for transplantation.

Previous thoracic surgery should be considered on an individual basis for each potential lung transplant recipient. In general, for single lung transplants, surgeons prefer the contralateral side to a previous thoracic surgical procedure. For bilateral lung transplants, acceptable previous procedures usually include open lung biopsies, chest tubes, tetracycline or bleomycin pleurodesis, or mechanical abrasion of the pleural surface.

Individuals with active or recent lung cancer are not eligible for lung transplantation.

Tobacco usage should not be tolerated. Many centers test potential candidates repeatedly for nicotine metabolites and reserve the right to remove candidates from the list if evidence of tobacco usage is found. Most centers have detected a return to smoking in a small percentage of patients after successful lung transplantation.

Optimal candidates for lung transplantation should not take chronic systemic corticosteroids, or, if clinically needed, the lowest dose possible should be prescribed. Most patients with well-defined advanced pulmonary emphysema derive little benefit from chronic systemic corticosteroids.

Candidates should be screened for skeletal muscle weakness and osteoporosis. Muscle weakness is most often related to steroid-induced myopathy, but hypoxemia, malnutrition, inactivity, and even testosterone deficiency play a contributory role.

Osteoporosis is extremely common in end-stage pulmonary disease (Shane et al 1996). In a study of 70 patients waiting for lung transplantation, osteoporosis T score below 2.5 was present in 30% of patients at the lumbar spine and 49% at the femoral neck, and osteopenia T score between 1 and

2.5 was present in an additional 35% of patients at the lumbar spine and 31% at the femoral neck. Only 34% of patients had normal bone density at the lumbar spine and only 22% had normal bone mass density at the hip. The average femoral neck T score of patients with emphysema (-2.7 ± 0.3) fell into the osteoporotic range, and was significantly below that of patients with other lung diseases (-1.5 ± 0.3), except for patients with cystic fibrosis (CF) (-2.6 ± 0.3). Duration of exposure to glucocorticoids correlated negatively with lumbar spine bone density. Most disturbing was the fact that very few patients were on sufficient regimens to prevent bone loss, and up to 20% of patients with emphysema were deficient in vitamin D. Osteoporosis should be treated aggressively before transplant to minimize risk of fracture after transplantation (Shane et al 1999).

Physiology of the Transplanted Lung

A general review of the physiology of the transplanted lung, including pulmonary denervation, impaired cough and mucociliary clearance, lymphatic interruption, vascular tone, and right ventricular function, has been recently published (Schulman 1998). This section will be limited to a discussion of aspects of lung transplantation specific to pulmonary emphysema.

Spirometry and lung volumes after lung transplantation have been well studied. Sequential spirometry measurements show a high degree of variability during the first postoperative year, due to increasing values for FVC and FEV_1. However, after the first postoperative year, variability in FVC and FEV_1 is less than 11% to 12%, and a decline in FVC and FEV_1 greater than 12% strongly suggests graft dysfunction due to infection or rejection (Martinez et al 1997).

Most bilateral lung transplant recipients achieve normal static and dynamic lung volumes with resolution of thoracic hyperinflation (Arens et al 1998). In addition, FRC and RV return to normal (Tamm et al 1994, Guignon et al 1995). These findings are in contrast to data in patients with CF who demonstrate a persistent increase in FRC and RV even after transplant, related to persistent over-inflation of the chest wall due to rib cage expansion along the anteroposterior diameter (Guignon et al). The difference between pulmonary emphysema and CF may relate to the fact that most of the hyperinflation in emphysema involves downward displacement of the diaphragm (Guignon et al). Since emphysema develops in adulthood, the rib cage is not substantially deformed. In contrast, patients with CF develop the disease in childhood, when the bony rib cage is still growing and can be remodeled considerably (Guignon et al). Since changes in thoracic structure in patients with pulmonary emphysema are reversible, it is most appropriate to use the recipient's *predicted* lung volumes as the normal values after transplantation, and the best method of matching donor and recipient volumes is to use their respective predicted TLC values (Tamm et al).

Aside from spirometry and lung volumes, other parameters of respiratory function after bilateral lung transplantation for pulmonary emphysema are remarkably intact: there is no evidence of airflow obstruction (normal FEV_1/FVC, normal airway resistance) (Arens et al 1998); distribution of alveolar ventilation (measured by single breath N2 washout) is normal; muscle pressures are normal; pulmonary arterial pressures are normal; gas exchange is normal at rest and with exercise; and the resting breathing pattern is no different from normal subjects.

In contrast to bilateral lung transplants, pulmonary function in single lung transplant recipients is highly dependent on physiologic interactions with the diseased native lung. In the immediate postoperative period, there may be acute mediastinal shift secondary to overdistention of the native emphysematous lung, with impaired gas exchange and even impaired hemodynamics. To minimize mediastinal shift in patients with pulmonary emphysema, transplant surgeons prefer to implant an "oversized" lung. Later in the postoperative course, the transplant lung usually appears radiographically "smaller" than the native, hyperinflated lung. In one study, the volume of the transplant lung was only 33% of TLC, whereas the volume of the native emphysema lung was 75% to 80% of TLC (Cheriyan et al 1995).

Despite these volume discrepancies, there is marked clinical improvement. Spirometry and arterial oxygen tension rapidly improve, and lung function continues to improve during the first postoperative year. In one study, at 12 months after single lung transplantation, mean FEV_1 increased from 0.49 (16% predicted) to 1.6 (54% predicted), FVC increased from 1.7 (43% predicted) to 2.4 (62% predicted), and FEV_1/FVC rose from 0.3 to 0.62 (Levine et al 1994). Mean PaO_2 increased from 58 mm Hg to 90 mm Hg, and no patient required supplemental oxygen at rest or exercise. Quantitative ventilation and perfusion to the transplant lung were 84% and 80%, respectively. These improvements were sustained during the second year after transplant.

There do not appear to be significant differences in physiologic parameters in patients undergoing right versus left single lung transplantation for emphysema (Levine et al 1994). A biphasic pattern of expiratory flow is often observed in the flow-volume curve (Herlihy et al 1994). The initial high-flow phase of the flow-volume curve derives from the transplanted lung, and the terminal low-flow from the native, emphysematous lung.

However, despite the improvement in airflow obstruction after single lung transplantation, the thorax remains hyperinflated, with TLC ranging from 110% to 120% predicted (Cheriyan et al 1995, Estenne et al 1999). Maximal inspiratory muscle pressures and maximal negative pleural pressures at TLC remain reduced (Cheriyan et al). As noted before, TLC on the transplanted side remains considerably smaller than TLC on the native side (Cheriyan et al, Estenne et al). In contrast, FRC on the transplanted side is normal despite elevated FRC on the native side. These findings are best explained by reduced inspiratory muscle generating capacity (either inspiratory muscle weakness or inspiratory muscles operating at shorter than optimal length due to persistent thoracic hyperinflation).

Risks and Benefits of Lung Transplantation

Evaluating risks and benefits of lung transplantation for pulmonary emphysema requires weighing the dramatic gains in pulmonary function against postoperative survival and complications. Early postoperative mortality for all lung transplant recipients is 7% to 10% and the 1-year survival rate is approximately 75% (Hosenpud et al 1999). The average survival rate after lung transplantation is 3.8 years.

Remarkably, patients with pulmonary emphysema fare better after lung transplantation than other diagnosis groups (Hosenpud et al 1999). In multivariate logistic regression analysis, a diagnosis of pulmonary emphysema reduced the risk ratio of 1-year mortality after lung transplantation by 52%. One-year survival rates as high as 90% to 92% have been reported after single and bilateral lung transplantation for pulmonary emphysema (Gaissert et al 1996). Some centers have reported better survival results after bilateral lung transplantation (1-year survival 90%) than after single lung transplantation (1-year survival 71%) (Bavaria et al 1997). Two-year survival rates after lung transplantation for pulmonary emphysema decline to 82% to 90% for bilateral lung transplant recipients and 63% to 84% for single lung transplant recipients (Bavaria et al, Sundaresan et al 1996). Five-year survival rates drop as low as 41% to 53% (Sundaresan et al). There have been no major changes in survival rates in the past few years (Hosenpud et al).

In view of the perioperative and later postoperative mortality risks for lung transplantation, some investigators have questioned whether there is a survival benefit associated with lung transplantation in the treatment of advanced pulmonary emphysema. Hosenpud and colleagues used UNOS data to compare survival curves for patients waiting for lung transplantation and for those after transplantation (Hosenpud et al 1998). Strictly speaking, these survival curves cannot be statistically compared; therefore, the authors generated a model to estimate relative risk of death from lung transplantation relative to the risk of continued waiting while on the transplant waiting list. For all diagnoses, the relative risk was high immediately after transplantation, reflecting perioperative mortality associated with transplant surgery. For patients with CF and idiopathic pulmonary fibrosis, the relative risk of transplant soon dropped below the risk of waiting, reflecting high mortality associated with the continued waiting. However, for patients with pulmonary emphysema, the relative risk of transplant never dropped below the risk of waiting, reflecting stable mortality rates associated with continued waiting while on the transplant waiting list.

The data raise serious concerns regarding survival benefits of lung transplantation in the treatment of advanced pulmonary emphysema. The data, however, are flawed in a basic premise. The analysis assumed that all patients with pulmonary emphysema listed for lung transplant were sick enough to need transplant surgery at the time of listing. Given the long waiting time for lung transplantation, many centers may "list" a patient for transplant in anticipation of need at the end of the long waiting time. This unofficial policy would bias results in favor of waiting list survival.

These considerations highlight a major dilemma faced by transplant physicians and surgeons. On the one hand, guidelines for referring patients with pulmonary emphysema for transplantation are able to identify those at risk of death in subsequent years. However, the natural history of pulmonary emphysema is so variable that the exact *timing* of transplant surgery is difficult to define. Accordingly, transplant centers and the referring physicians rely on additional clinical criteria to determine the optimal timing for lung transplantation. Such criteria include rapid decline in pulmonary function, frequent exacerbations, and deteriorating gas exchange. Waiting too long to proceed with transplantation may cause patients to lose their suitability for transplantation by developing worsening debility or respiratory failure.

Another limitation of the analysis by Hosenpud et al was that the data assessed the duration of survival but not the quality of life. After successful lung transplantation, there are dramatic improvements in the health and quality of life of the patient. One study of transplant recipients reported higher levels of happiness, more satisfaction with life and health, better function on the Karnofsky index, and higher levels in every MOS 20 dimension except pain (Gross et al 1995). Furthermore, health-related quality of life remained stable 3 years after transplantation, although there was some decline over time in patients who developed chronic rejection. Between 85% to 90% of lung transplant recipients reported no activity limitation at 1 and 2 years after transplant (Hosenpud et al 1999).

Despite improved pulmonary function and quality of life, transplant recipients face numerous postoperative complications (Trulock 1997, Arcasoy and Kotloff 1999). One-half of transplant recipients required repeat hospitalization during the first year after transplantation (Hosenpud et al 1999). Postoperative morbidities may be conveniently divided into respiratory and nonrespiratory issues. In the perioperative period, respiratory complications include ischemia-reperfusion injury, bronchial anastomotic complications (ischemia, dehiscence, stenosis), pulmonary vein thrombosis, and pneumonia. Unique to single lung transplantation for pulmonary emphysema is acute mediastinal shift with hypoxemia and hypotension. This is best managed with independent lung ventilation to deliberately underventilate the native emphysematous lung to prevent hyperinflation, while maintaining normal ventilation parameters to the transplanted lung.

Later postoperative respiratory complications include acute rejection, opportunistic infection, and chronic rejection (Bando et al 1995, Sharples et al 1996). Acute allograft rejection, characterized by perivascular lymphocytic inflammation, is common, rarely fatal, and tends to respond favorably to augmented immunosuppression. In contrast, obliterative bronchiolitis (OB), which is generally considered to represent chronic allograft rejection, is characterized by fibrous obliteration of small airways, responds poorly to augmented immunosuppression, and is the major cause of long-term morbidity and mortality after lung transplantation. A number of studies have identified multiple and high-grade acute rejection episodes as the major risk factors for OB, yet the pathogenetic mechanisms linking acute perivascular rejection to chronic airway obliteration remain undefined. These complications occur at similar rates for patients transplanted for pulmonary emphysema as compared with patients transplanted for other diagnoses.

Unique to single lung transplantation for pulmonary emphysema is native lung hyperinflation with compression and atelectasis of the allograft. Other problems fairly specific to single lung transplantation for pulmonary emphysema are potential diseases related to the native lung. These include pneumothorax, bronchogenic carcinoma, reactivation of dormant tuberculous and nontuberculous mycobacterial infections, and contamination of the transplant lung with pathogens such as gram negative bacteria and aspergillus.

Nonrespiratory complications after lung transplantation are numerous and include systemic hypertension, renal insufficiency, diabetes mellitus, hyperlipidemia, seizures, osteoporosis, gastroparesis, and posttransplant lymphoproliferative disorder. Most nonrespiratory complications are related directly, or indirectly, to adverse effects of transplant medications.

References

The Alpha 1-Antitrypsin Deficiency Registry Study Group. 1995. Survival and FEV$_1$ decline in individuals with severe deficiency of alpha 1-antitrypsin. *Am J Respir Crit Care Med.* 151:369-373.

Anthonisen, NR. 1989. Prognosis in chronic obstructive pulmonary disease: results from multicenter clinical trials. *Am Rev Respir Dis.* 140:S95-S99.

Arcasoy, SM and RM Kotloff. 1999. Lung transplantation. *N Engl J Med.* 340:1081-1091.

Arens, R, JM McDonough, H Zhao, NP Blumenthal, RM Kotloff, and MM Grunstein. 1998. Altered lung mechanics after double-lung transplantation. *Am J Respir Crit Care Med.* 158:1403-1409.

Bando, K, IL Paradis, S Similo et al. 1995. Obliterative bronchiolitis after lung and heart-lung transplantation: an analysis of risk factors and management. *J Thorac Cardiovasc Surg.* 110:4-14.

Bavaria, JE, R Kotloff, H Palevsky et al. 1997. Bilateral versus single lung transplantation for chronic obstructive pulmonary disease. *J Thorac Cardiovasc Surg.* 113:520-528.

Cheriyan, AF, ER Garrity, R Pifarre, PJ Fahey, and JM Walsh. 1995. Reduced transplant lung volumes after single lung transplantation for chronic obstructive pulmonary disease. *Am J Respir Crit Care Med.* 151:851-853.

Cooper, JD. 1997. The history of surgical procedures for emphysema. *Ann Thorac Surg.* 63:312-319.

Estenne, M, M Cassart, P Poncelet, and PA Gevenois. 1999. Volume of graft and native lung after single-lung transplantation for emphysema. *Am J Respir Crit Care Med.* 159:641-645.

Gaissert, HA, EP Trulock, JD Cooper, RS Sundaresan, and GA Patterson. 1996. Comparison of early functional results after volume reduction or lung transplantation for chronic obstructive pulmonary disease. *J Thorac Cardiovasc Surg.* 111:296-307.

Gray-Donald, K, L Gibbons, SH Shapiro, PT Macklem, and JG Martin. 1996. Nutritional status and mortality in chronic obstructive pulmonary disease. *Am J Respir Crit Care Med.* 153:961-966.

Gross, CR, K Savik, RM Bolman, and MI Hertz. 1995. Long-term health status and quality of life outcomes of lung transplant recipients. *Chest.* 108:1587-1593.

Guignon I, M Cassart, PA Gevenois et al. 1995. Persistent hyperinflation after heart-lung transplantation for cystic fibrosis. *Am J Respir Crit Care Med.* 151:534-540.

Herlihy JP, JG Venegas, DM Systrom et al. 1994. Expiratory flow pattern following single-lung transplantation in emphysema. *Am J Respir Crit Care Med.* 150:1684-1689.

Hosenpud JD, LE Bennett, BM Keck, B Fiol, MM Boucek, and RJ Novick. 1999. The registry of the International Society for Heart and Lung Transplantation: sixteenth official report. *J Heart Lung Transplant.* 18:611-626.

Hosenpud JD, LE Bennett, BM Keck, EB Edwards, and RJ Novick. 1998. Effect of diagnosis on survival benefit of lung transplantation for end-stage lung disease. *Lancet.* 351:24-27.

Joint statement of the American Society for Transplant Physicians, American Thoracic Society, European Respiratory Society, and International Society for Heart and Lung Transplantation. 1998. International guidelines for the selection of lung transplant candidates. *Am J Respir Crit Care Med.* 158:335-339.

Levine, SM, A Anzueto, JI Peters et al. 1994. Medium term functional results of single-lung transplantation for endstage obstructive lung disease. *Am J Respir Crit Care Med.* 150:398-402.

Martinez, JA, IL Paradis, JH Dauber et al. 1997. Spirometry values in stable lung transplant recipients. *Am J Respir Crit Care Med.* 155:285-290.

Nash, ES, WA Briscoe, and A Cournand. 1965. The relationship between clinical and physiological findings in chronic obstructive disease of the lungs. *Med Thorac.* 22:305-327.

Schulman, LL. 1998. Physiology of the transplanted lung. In *Primer on Transplantation*, eds. Norman and Suki, 519-526. Chelsea, MI: Slack Inc.

Schulman, LL, PP Lennon, JA Wood, and Y Enson. 1994. Pulmonary vascular resistance in emphysema. *Chest.* 105:798-805.

Shane, E, A Papadopoulos, RB Staron et al. 1999. Bone loss and fracture after lung transplantation. *Transplantation.* 68:220-227.

Shane, E, SJ Silverberg, D Donovan et al. 1996. Osteoporosis in lung transplantation candidates with end-stage pulmonary disease. *Am J Med.* 101:262-269.

Sharples, LD, M Tamm, K McNeil, TW Higenbottam, Stewart, and J Wallwork. 1996. Development of bronchiolitis obliterans syndrome in recipients of heart-lung transplantation: early risk factors. *Transplantation*. 61:560-566.

Stevens, PM, PC Johnson, RL Bell, AC Beall, and DE Jenkins. 1970. Regional ventilation and perfusion after lung transplantation in patients with emphysema. *N Engl J Med*. 282:245-249.

Sundaresan, RS, Y Shiraishi, EP Trulock et al. 1996. Single or bilateral lung transplantation for emphysema? *J Thorac Cardiovasc Surg*. 112:1485-1495.

Tamm, M, TW Higenbottam, CM Dennis, LD Sharples, and J Wallwork. 1994. Donor and recipient predicted lung volume and lung size after heart-lung transplantation. *Am J Respir Crit Care Med*. 150: 403-407.

Toronto Lung Transplant Group. 1988. Experience with single-lung transplantation for pulmonary fibrosis. *JAMA*. 259:2258-2262.

Trulock, EP. 1997. Lung transplantation. *Am J Respir Crit Care Med*. 155:789-818.

7

Lung Volume Reduction Surgery and the National Emphysema Treatment Trial

Byron M. Thomashow, MD

Chronic obstructive pulmonary disease (COPD) is now the fourth leading cause of death in this country, and the only major disease continuing to increase in prevalence and mortality (National Center for Health Statistics 1993). There are over 20 million people in this country with COPD (Celli et al 1995, Adam et al 1992). Most of these have the asthmatic or chronic bronchitic forms of the disease, but many are felt to have the emphysematous type. While asthma and chronic bronchitis tend to be medically treatable and medically controllable diseases, there is no good medical therapy for emphysema (Burrows et al 1987). Disability is the exception in asthma and chronic bronchitis; it is the rule in progressive emphysema. Also, in studies comparing mortality risks, 10-year mortality is far higher in emphysema than in the asthmatic or chronic bronchitic groups (Hodgkin 1990).

Because medical therapy has been so limited in emphysema, for over 100 years medicine has looked for surgical options. During that time, many procedures have been attempted. Most appeared promising initially, only to be abandoned because of ineffectiveness, morbidity, or mortality risks (Knudson and Gaensler 1965, Foreman et al 1968, American Thoracic Society 1968, Fitzgerald et al 1974). Over the last decade, single lung transplantation has been successfully performed in patients with severe emphysema, but lung transplantation remains very expensive, and many problems persist, including infection, rejection, and bronchiolitis obliterans.

Lung Volume Reduction Surgery

In 1993, Dr. Joel Cooper reintroduced a surgical procedure initially performed by Dr. Otto Brantigan in the 1950s (Brantigan and Mueller 1957, Brantigan et al 1959) in which the worse areas of emphysematous lung were removed. Dr. Cooper published some very encouraging results (Cooper et al 1995). Subsequently, this procedure, lung volume reduction surgery (LVRS), was performed in a number of centers around the country. Published reports from numerous centers suggested that LVRS may be beneficial in selected emphysema patients (Argenziano et al 1996; Yusen,

Trulock et al 1996; McKenna, Brenner, Gelb et al 1996; Bingisser et al 1996).

At Columbia Presbyterian Medical Center (CPMC) in New York City, physicians followed Dr Cooper's lead. Dr. Cooper's work suggested that patients were more likely to benefit from LVRS if computerized axial tomography (CAT) scanning and perfusion lung scanning suggested heterogeneous disease, with so-called "target" areas with worse emphysema. Patients with significant chronic bronchitic or asthmatic components were excluded, as were patients with other medical problems, including significant cardiac disease.

In Dr. Cooper's 1995 publication, the standard for future evaluation of patients for LVRS was established (Cooper et al 1995). Dr. Cooper's patients underwent standard spirometry prebronchodilators and postbronchodilators, lung volumes by body plethysmography and nitrogen washout, standardized 6-minute walks, and arterial blood gas (ABG) studies. Radiographic evaluation included inspiratory and expiratory chest radiographs, CAT scanning, and quantitative nuclear perfusion and ventilation lung scanning. Patients completed quality of life assessments and dyspnea indices. All patients underwent right heart catheterizations. It is to Dr. Cooper's credit that more than 5 years after completing this initial study, the evaluation of patients for LVRS has remained basically unchanged. Of the evaluation described in the 1995 study, only nitrogen washout, ventilatory radionuclear scanning, and right heart catheterizations are no longer felt to be part of routine LVRS evaluations.

At CPMC, the initial 152 patients undergoing LVRS had an average age of 64 years. Fifty-four percent were female. Fifty-three percent were oxygen-dependent. Thirty-two percent had significant elevations of their partial pressure of carbon dioxide ($PaCO_2 > 45$ mm Hg). Eighty-two percent had forced expiratory volume in one second (FEV_1) less than 30% predicted. Forty percent of the patients had FEV_1 less than 20% predicted. The mean FEV_1 was 587 ± 223 cc. The mean forced vital capacity (FVC) was 1725 ± 639 cc. The total lung volume (TLC) averaged 7.2 ± 1.6 liters (over 150% predicted), and the residual volume (RV) averaged 5.25 ± 1.5 liters (over 200% predicted). Their dyspnea indices suggested that most of these patients became short of breath changing their clothes, and many were short of breath at rest. These were severely limited patients.

Unlike Dr. Cooper, who almost always performed LVRS bilaterally via a median sternotomy approach, surgeons at CPMC attempted to adjust the surgical approach to the anatomy of the patient's emphysema. Of the initial 152 patients, 93 underwent sternotomies with bilateral resections. However, because of concern over potential sternal dehiscence in those patients on significant steroid dosing, 46 of these patients underwent an inframammary approach, the so-called "clamshell" procedure where less of the sternum is cut. Fifty-four additional patients underwent unilateral procedures either via thoracotomy or thoracoscopy. Most of these had had prior contralateral lung surgery, prior contralateral pleural or parenchymal disease, or suspicious lung nodules. A small number of patients underwent staged thoracoscopic procedures.

In the CPMC experience, there was a significant increase in FEV_1, averaging over 200 cc, which generally persisted over a 3-year follow-up period. In those patients who underwent bilateral procedures, the improvement in FEV_1 was even higher, averaging 61%. This figure is similar to other reported improvements (Yusen, Trulock et al 1996; McKenna, Brenner, Gelb et al 1996; Bingisser et al 1996). All studies have shown a greater benefit with bilateral LVRS compared with a unilateral approach (McKenna, Brenner, Fischal et al 1996; Argenziano et al 1997), and this has been the CPMC experience as well. After LVRS, CPMC patients were found to have a significant reduction in RV, averaging over 2 liters, and this improvement in most patients appeared to persist over a 3-year period. Even more marked than the improvements in pulmonary function studies was a dramatic improvement in the quality of life and sensation of dyspnea in most patients. Many patients had a significant decrease in oxygen requirements after surgery, although these requirements gradually increased again over the 1- to 2-year postsurgery period.

Why LVRS works when it works, and why it fails when it fails, remains somewhat unclear. Gelb et al have shown significant improvement in lung elastic recoil after LVRS (1997). While this improvement decreases over the following 2 years, it remains better than baseline. Other investigators have shown improvement in airflow limitation (Fessler and Permutt 1998), improvement in diaphragmatic strength (Criner et al 1998), and improvement in lung and chest wall mechanics (Bernas et al 1998). The CPMC group has published data showing that a decrease in lung volumes on CAT scanning correlated with improvements in pulmonary function testing (Becker et al 1998). In addition, by using quantitative CAT scanning techniques these investigators were able to show an increase in denser, more normal-appearing lung tissue, suggesting that expansion of "better" lung tissue, presumably previously compressed by over-expanded emphysematous lung, may play a role in postoperative improvement.

Some investigators have suggested that LVRS may improve pulmonary hemodynamics (Wex et al 1983). However, this is an area of considerable concern to pulmonologists and surgeons caring for potential LVRS candidates (Kubo et al 1998, Oswald-Mammoser et al 1998, Weg et al 1999). Many patients with severe emphysema have mild to moderate pulmonary hypertension. Even though surgeons attempt to remove those lung areas with decreased perfusion as indicated on CAT and perfusion lung scanning, some capillary bed has to be resected, therefore potentially increasing pulmonary hypertension. Some of the deaths after LVRS have been felt to be secondary to this increased pulmonary hypertension.

Indeed, as impressive as the initial CPMC results have been and as well as they have correlated with other published results, it must be stressed that the surgery does carry significant risk. There is significant morbidity. In the CPMC experience, 42% of patients had prolonged air leaks requiring chest tubes for over 2 weeks. Seven percent required prolonged ventilatory dependence, 3% had cardiovascular events, and another 1% had gastrointestinal complications. These complications contributed to a prolonged length of hospital stay. At CPMC, the average length of stay was 25 days for the first 51 patients, 17 days for the next 51 patients, and 12 days for the next 50 patients. As physicians have become more experienced with both selection criteria and perioperative care, length of stay has continued to fall. More recently, patients at most centers have a length of stay less than 7 to 10 days.

In addition to morbidity risks, LVRS carries significant mortality risks. In the CPMC experience, 8 of the first 75 patients died within 3 months of surgery. As experience increased, mortality rates decreased. At CPMC, only 3 the next 77 patients died within the first 3 postoperative months. These early deaths included a cerebrovascular accident, a myocardial infarction, a gastrointestinal hemorrhage, several pulmonary emboli, and several felt most likely to be secondary to increased pulmonary hypertension. In addition to these early postoperative deaths, 25 other patients undergoing LVRS at CPMC died between 1 and 3 years after surgery. Most of these late deaths have been secondary to respiratory failure from progressive emphysema. Even with these deaths, Kaplan Meier curves have suggested a 4-year estimated mortality of 30% in patients after LVRS, which correlates well with historical models of similar patients with severe emphysema. In addition, if patients over the age of 70 and patients with elevated PCO_2 are eliminated [these groups have been shown to have higher mortality in other studies as well (Brenner et al 1996, 1999; Keenan et al 1996; Yusen et al 1996)], mortality curves appear more favorable.

National Emphysema Treatment Trial

In addition to problems with morbidity and mortality, and concerns as to how long benefits persist when they do occur, there are potential data problems with most of the published studies of LVRS. Most of the studies have relatively short follow-up data, have incomplete follow-up, use average data, and lack significant quality of life information. Because of these data concerns, in 1995 Medicare suspended coverage for LVRS and the procedure is now the subject of a multicenter randomized 7-year National Institutes of Health study, the National Emphysema Treatment Trial (NETT). This study should determine relative risks and benefits of the procedure and outline selection criteria. Ultimately, these selection criteria should allow better definition of the evaluation process for potential LVRS candidates.

The evaluation of patients for LVRS can be broadly divided into 3 areas: clinical status, pulmonary function evaluation, and radiographic assessment. The evaluation of potential LVRS candidates starts with a complete history, physical examination, and routine laboratory studies. Important clinical issues include patient age, smoking history, bronchitic component, nutritional status, level of disability, extent of systemic steroid requirements, cardiac status, presence of pulmonary hypertension, presence of other significant lung diseases, and presence of other significant medical diseases. Pulmonary function evaluation includes spirometry prebronchodilators and postbronchodilators, lung volumes, and ABG measurements. Radiographic studies include inspiratory/expiratory chest radiographs, CAT scanning, and perfusion lung scanning. Evaluation includes echocardiogram and dobutamine radionucleide cardiac scanning, and cardiopulmonary exercise testing. Potential candidates complete 6-minute walks and undergo quality of life evaluations. NETT patients undergo these screening studies over a 3 to 4-day period of outpatient evaluation.

In the NETT, inclusion criteria include a history and physical examination consistent with emphysema, CAT scan evidence of bilateral emphysema, a TLC greater than 100% predicted, an RV greater than 150% predicted, an FEV_1 less than 45% predicted, and a postbronchodilator increase in FEV_1 less than 30% or 300 ml. In addition, because of prior experience performing LVRS in patients over age 70 (Brenner et al 1996, 1999), these patients must have an FEV_1 greater than 15% predicted. NETT candidates must have a $PaCO_2$ less than 61 mm Hg. The NETT also requires a room air resting PaO_2 equal to or greater than 45 mm Hg and oxygen requirements during rest or with oxygen titration not exceeding 6 l/min to keep saturation over 90%. Higher oxygen requirements reflect either the severity of the underlying emphysema, suggesting little remaining functional lung tissue, or the presence of another lung problem in addition to the emphysema. In either case, LVRS would likely be of little benefit and operative risks would be high.

NETT candidates must be nonsmokers for at least 4 months prior to evaluation. Patients must have plasma cotinine levels under 13.7 ng/ml if not using preventive nicotine products, or an arterial carboxyhemoglobin under 2.5% if using preventive nicotine products. In addition, males must have a body mass index less than 31.2 kg/m^2 and females less than 32.4 kg/m^2.

Approval for surgery by a cardiologist is required in the NETT if patients have unstable angina, a left ventricular ejection fraction under 45%, a dobutamine radionucleide cardiac scan indicating coronary artery disease or ventricular dysfunction, more than 5 premature ventricular beats per minute, cardiac arrhythmia, or an S3 gallop on examination.

Exclusion criteria in the NETT include evidence of a systemic disease or neoplasia likely to compromise survival over the duration of the trial, previous LVRS, previous sternotomy or lobectomy, clinically significant bronchiectasis, or a pulmonary nodule requiring surgery. Patients with giant bulla (greater than 1/3 of the volume of that lung) or significant pleural or interstitial disease are also excluded. While diffuse homogeneous emphysema is not a contraindication, most surgeons have been reluctant to include patients who appear to have little functioning lung tissue on scanning.

Other NETT exclusion criteria include a history of a myocardial infarction or congestive heart failure within 6 months if the left ventricular ejection fraction remains less than 45%, uncontrolled hypertension with systolic pressures over 200 mm Hg or diastolic pressures over 110 mm Hg, or unplanned recent weight loss over 10% of usual weight. If, on echocardiogram, peak systolic pulmonary artery pressures are estimated to be greater than 44 mm Hg, a right heart catheterization is mandatory. If, on right heart catheterization, mean pulmonary artery pressures are greater than 34 mm Hg or peak systolic pressures are greater than 44 mm Hg, patients are excluded. Because of concern over potential steroid complications, patients requiring over 20 mg of Prednisone or equivalent are also excluded.

If patients meet the NETT criteria and sign appropriate consents, they then enter a period of intensive pulmonary rehabilitation. This begins with 4 days of core rehabilitation at one of the 17 NETT centers and is completed with 6 to 8 weeks of rehabilitation either at the centers or at satellite centers certified by the NETT. Once the pulmonary rehabilitation period is completed, patients are reevaluated at the core centers. They repeat pulmonary function studies, 6-minute walks, quality of life forms, and cardiopulmonary exercise testing. If they are still candidates, and if they formally consent, they are then randomized to either surgery or medical groups. Depending on the center, the surgery could be performed either by a median sternotomy or a bilateral video assisted thoracoscopic (VATS) approach. All patients in both medical and surgical groups resume and continue pulmonary rehabilitation. NETT patients must return to the centers for regular follow-up, which includes repeated pulmonary function studies, cardiopulmonary exercise testing, 6-minute walks, and quality of life assessments.

It is expected that the NETT will clarify the potential role of LVRS in the treatment of emphysematous patients, the efficacy of LVRS compared with medical therapy, and the efficacy of LVRS by median sternotomy vs. VATS. The NETT results should also better define selection criteria for LVRS and provide a cost-effectiveness analysis comparing LVRS with maximal medical therapy. Whatever the final results of the NETT, and whatever the ultimate role of LVRS in emphysema patients, one would have to believe that attempting to prevent the development of emphysema by decreasing cigarette use remains our long-term best hope.

References

Adam, RF and V Benson. 1992. Current estimates from the National Health Interview Survey, 1991. National Center for Health Statistics. *Vital Health Stat.* 10(184).

American Thoracic Society. 1968. Current status of the surgical treatment of pulmonary emphysema and asthma. *Am Rev Respir Dis.* 97:486-489.

Argenziano, M, N Mozami, B Thomashow et al. 1996. Extended indications for volume reduction pneumectomy in advanced emphysema. *J Thorac Cardiovasc Surg.* 62:1588-1597.

Argenziano, M, B Thomashow, P Jellen et al. 1997. A functional comparison of unilateral vs. bilateral lung volume reduction surgery. *Ann Thorac Surg.* 64:321-327.

Becker, M, Y Berkman, J Austin et al. 1998. Lung volumes before and after lung volume reduction surgery: quantitative CT analysis. *Am J Respir Crit Care Med.* 157:1593-1599.

Bernas, G, T Gilbert, M Krasna et al. 1998. Acute effects of bilateral lung volume reduction surgery on lung and chest wall mechanical properties. *Chest.* 11:61-68.

Bingisser, R, A Zollinger, M Hauser et al. 1996. Bilateral volume reduction surgery for diffuse pulmonary emphysema by video assisted thoracoscopy. *J Thorac Cardiovasc Surg.* 112:875-882.

Brantigan, O and E Mueller. 1957. Surgical treatment of pulmonary emphysema. *Am Surg.* 23:789-804.

Brantigan, O, E Mueller, and M Kress. 1959. A surgical approach to pulmonary emphysema. *Am Rev Respir Dis.* 80:194-202.

Brenner, M, R McKenna, J Chen et al. 1999. Survival following bilateral staple lung reduction surgery for emphysema. *Chest.* 115:390-396.

Brenner, M, R Yusen, and R McKenna. 1996. Lung volume reduction surgery for emphysema. *Chest.* 110:205-218.

Burrows, B, JW Bloom, GA Traver et al. 1987. The course and prognosis of different forms of chronic airways obstruction in a sample from the general population. *N Eng J Med.* 317:1309-1314.

Celli, BR, GL Snider, J Heffner et al. 1995. Standards for the diagnosis and care of patients with COPD. *Am J Respir Crit Care Med.* 152 (Suppl 5):S78-121.

Cooper, J, E Trulock, A Triantafillou et al. 1995. Bilateral pneumectomy (volume reduction) for chronic obstructive pulmonary disease. *J Thorac Cardiovasc Surg.* 109:106-119.

Criner, G, F Cordova, V Levenson et al. 1998. Effect of lung volume reduction surgery on diaphragm strength. *Am J Respir Crit Care Med.* 157:1578-1585.

Fessler, H and S Permutt. 1998. Lung volume reduction surgery an airflow limitation. *Am J Respir Crit Care Med.* 157:715-722.

Fitzgerald, M, P Keelan, D Cagell et al. 1974. Long-term results of surgery for bullous emphysema. *J Thorac Cardiovasc Surg.* 65:566-587.

Foreman, S, H Weil, R Duke et al. 1968. Bullous disease of the lungs: physiologic improvement after surgery. *Ann Intern Med.* 69:757-767.

Gelb, A, M Brenner, R McKeon et al. 1997. Serial lung function and elastic recoil two years after lung volume reduction surgery for emphysema. *Chest.* 111:550-558.

Hodgkin, J. 1990. Prognosis in chronic obstructive pulmonary disease. *Clinics in Chest Med.* 11(3):555-569.

Keenan, R, R Landreneau, F Sciurba et al. 1996. Unilateral thoracoscopic surgical approach for diffuse emphysema. *J Thorac Cardiovasc Surg.* 112:208-216.

Knudson, R and E Gaensler. 1965. Surgery for emphysema. *Ann Thorac Surg.* 1:332-362.

Kubo, K, T Koizami, K Fujimoto et al. 1998. Effects of lung volume reduction surgery on exercise pulmonary hemodynamics in severe emphysema. *Chest.* 114:1575-1582.

McKenna, R, M Brenner, R Fischal et al. 1996. Should lung volume reduction be unilateral or bilateral? *J Thorac Cardiovasc Surg.* 112:1331-1339.

McKenna, RJ, M Brenner, AF Gelb et al. 1996. A randomized prospective trial of stapled lung reduction versus laser bullectomy for diffuse emphysema. *J Thorac Cardiovasc Surg.* 111:317-321.

National Center for Health Statistics. 1993. *Advance Report of Final Mortality Statistics 1991.* Monthly vital statistics report. Suppl. 42(2).

Oswald-Mammoser, M, R Kessler, G Massard et al. 1998. Effect of lung volume reduction surgery on gas exchanges and pulmonary hemodynamics at rest and during exercise. *Am J Respir Crit Care Med.* 158:1020-1025.

Weg, I, L Rossoff, K McKeon et al. 1999. Development of pulmonary hypertension after lung volume reduction surgery. *Am J Respir Crit Care Med.* 159:552-556.

Wex, P, H Ebner, and D Dragojevic. 1983. Functional surgery of bullous emphysema. *Thorac Cardiovasc Surg.* 31:346-351.

Yusen, R and S Lefrak. 1996. Evaluation of patients with emphysema for lung volume reduction surgery. *Semin Thorac Cardiovasc Surg.* 8:83-93.

Yusen, R, E Trulock, M Pohl et al. 1996. Results of lung volume reduction surgery in patients with emphysema. *Semin Thorac Cardiovasc Surg.* 8:99-109.

8

Marital Stress and Coping With A1AD Emphysema

Christine A. Cannon, PhD, RN

The author's interest in the interaction between A1AD and marriage stems from a long history of professional and volunteer involvement with families coping with COPD. It is sustained by the many couples who so willingly have shared their personal lives to help others. One of the most powerful marital partnerships that she has had the pleasure of knowing is that of Richard and Evelyn Heering. After decades of living with A1AD, Richard died, leaving a void within the international A1AD community. Evelyn has continued as a mainstay of support to the many caregivers who struggle for their own survival.

Advancing chronic lung disease is fought on many fronts. When it is caused by an inherited deficiency of alpha 1-antitrypsin (A1AD), the lives of young, often middle-aged, men and women are forever changed. Their close relationships must rise to the challenges posed by the progressive loss of respiratory function. In order to provide palliative care as lung destruction advances, the effects of A1AD within the marriage—the context in which the illness is experienced and managed—must be considered. Health care providers can affect the quality of life in cases of advanced disease by providing support and information to couples from the time of diagnosis. Research conducted over the last 4 years suggests that marriages affected by A1AD that are "good," resilient, and empowering have a significantly positive impact on both partners—on their quality of life, their perceived competence in managing feelings, the frequency of depressive symptoms, and the severity of stress related to wheezing, coughing, and infections (Cannon 1997, 1999).

An ongoing multiphase study of marriages was begun in 1995 to gain insight into living with emphysema associated with A1AD. The purpose of the study is to describe the impact of this late-onset, genetic disorder on both spouses and on the relationship that they share, as well as analyze the responses within marriage that foster biopsychosocial well-being and the exchange of support. The results of three segments of the multiphase research will be summarized in this chapter:

- similarities and differences in perceived stress and coping between marriages subgrouped by the number of years since diagnosis
- changes in functioning in satisfying marriages over a period of 1 year
- comparisons in characteristics, functioning, coping, and outcomes between more and less satisfying marriages

Once the implications of A1AD as it affects the marital system are known, interventions to help reduce its devastating impact can be planned. While medical efforts are targeted to reducing the destruction of lung tissue, much work is also needed to help prevent the destruction of marriages.

The Investigational Model

To organize the inquiry, a model was designed that incorporated findings of qualitative research employing interviews and focus groups and several theories and models. These findings substantiated the need to study marriage as a subsystem and to incorporate the principles of the Family Systems Theory (Whitchurch 1993), such as holism, nonsummitivity, morphogenesis, and interdependence; the Interdependence Theory (Thibaut 1959), which focuses on the influence of one partner on the outcomes of the other partner; and the Cognitive Phenomenological Theory of Psychological Stress (Lazarus 1984), which interrelates stress and resource appraisals with coping strategies. These theories address the dyadic, interpersonal, and individual perspectives, respectively. Breathlessness and progressive physical, psychological, and social losses—the two primary stressors identified—affected the well, as well as the ill, spouse in different ways. The thoughts of each partner related to these stressors were associated with feelings and behaviors within the marital relationship, supporting the integration of the Systems Model of Family Stress (Burr 1994), the Process Model of Family Functioning (Steinhauer 1984), and the Contextual Model of Marital Interaction (Bradbury 1989) into the model design. The initial qualitative inquiry and these theories and models served as the foundation for creating the study's investigative framework. The Marital Coping in Chronic Illness model/framework enables the biopsychosocial study of marriage at multiple levels—individual (patient, well spouse), interpersonal (within relationship), and dyadic (as a marital system)—in four areas: characteristics, functioning, coping, and outcomes (Cannon 1997).

Methodology

The first phases of the study employed qualitative methods: focus groups as well as telephone and face-to-face interviews and a written survey taken 1 year after the focus groups were held. Hundreds of pages of transcribed qualitative data were thematically analyzed and categorized, using open coding technique as described in the use of grounded theory (Strauss 1990).

The quantitative data were collected using investigator-designed questions combined with well-established measures of individual and marital functioning, coping, and outcomes. Surveys of 91 marriages were completed independently by each spouse. The quantitative data were described (measures of central tendency) and subdivided using cluster analysis to represent couples in two clusters—more mutually satisfying marriages and less satisfying marriages. *T* testing distinguished differences between clusters and within marriages (paired *t* tests) in each cluster (Cannon 1997).

Comparisons of Marriages Based on Time Since Diagnosis

Married couples attending the 1995 annual National Alpha 1 Educational Conference were divided into two focus groups based on the length of time since diagnosis with A1AD. "More experienced" couples (three male patients and their well wives) had an average of 9 years since the disease was diagnosed, while the "less experienced" couples (three male patients and their wives and three female patients and their husbands) had an average of 5 years since diagnosis. Both of these groups were further subdivided into patient and well-spouse groups for a total of six focus groups (Cannon 1997).

Sample Description

This sample of 9 couples—18 expert informants—was representative of couples managing A1AD and willing to participate in research. The means for age (55-56 years) and completed years of education (1-2 years beyond high school), and the distribution of second marriages (33%) and gender (33% female patients and well husbands and 67% male patients and well wives) for the sample showed no statistically significant differences from a larger sample of 91 couples who had participated in the quantitative phase of the study in 1996. Mean age, age of symptom onset, age of diagnosis, and length of prediagnosis period (years between symptom onset and A1AD diagnosis), as well as the gender and racial distributions of the focus group sample, were similar to samples of patients studied by Brantly and associates (1988), Larrson (1978), and Stoller and associates (1994) (Cannon 1997).

Similarities Among Groups

Similarities between the groups with more time since diagnosis and the groups with less time were found in their descriptions of the gravity of their situations and the impact of A1AD on their marriages. The stress of breathlessness was described as "consuming," "pervasive," "intrusive," and "devastating." Common topics included:

(a) the long, symptomatic prediagnosis period; (b) uncertainty of medical support and physician knowledge; (c) the intensity of the personal and interpersonal struggles related to control and adjustment; (d) the need to maintain self-integrity; and (e) the importance and benefits of marital communication and collaboration to meet illness-marital needs. (Cannon 1998:5)

The two groups of patients discussed similarities in the depth of their revelations concerning A1AD stress. Members of both spouse groups felt very involved in caring for their spouses' physical and emotional health.

Husbands and wives spoke of their pain in watching their spouses' suffering, and feeling little control over the situation. They spoke of trying to maintain their own physical health and control over their emotional pain, as they worked to maintain their ill spouses' self-esteem in the face of increasing dependence. Discussions of other family members' responses and the importance of faith occurred in both groups. (Cannon 1998:5)

Differences Between Groups

Couples with a longer time since A1AD diagnosis reflected on the past, present, and future of their illness-marriage trajectory. The patients in this group emphasized the loss of their physical capabilities, including work-related losses, yet they expressed acceptance of their increasing dependence on their families and of their anticipated decline, decisions, and death. Their well spouses (wives) expressed acceptance of the work of caregiving. In contrast, couples with a shorter period of time since diagnosis dwelled on the trauma surrounding their recent, yet delayed, diagnosis. They spent much time discussing the value of information gathering and sharing (Cannon 1997).

Those patients with more time since A1AD diagnosis compared their many experiences with breathlessness, related fears, and losses. They expressed the terror of not being able to breathe, the fear of being alone, the anxiety of claustrophobia, and the snowballing of panic. They focused on their future needs, decisions (such as transplantation), and their fate. Interestingly, the well wives of these patients expressed anger about being taken for granted and being limited in their life choices. In contrast, the patients with less time since diagnosis discussed their limitations and needs more broadly. They focused on their past successes, and optimism and positive comments were expressed much more frequently (Cannon 1997).

Changes in Marriages One Year Later

One year after the couples met in focus groups, all partners were interviewed to identify how their relationships had changed with time. In addition, they independently responded to "short answer" surveys. A summary follows of some of the findings that may be helpful in understanding relationship functioning and support.

Follow-up Interviews

Follow-up interviews revealed that all but two of the couples became closer over the intervening year. In fact, the stress of health changes in the partner with A1AD was perceived to have increased the level of marital satisfaction in several of the couples. In the two couples who became less satisfied with their relationships, the issue of the amount of time together was a stressor. In one of the marriages, the well wife was distressed over the decreasing amount of time she had with her ill husband, who spent his time working and sleeping to recover for the next day's work. The dramatic decrease in time together for recreation and leisure led to increasing depression and unhappiness. The well wife in the other couple suffered from having too much time for her husband's increasing dependency. One of these couples described feeling increasing interpersonal tension, a loss of openness, and being "out of sync" (Cannon 1997).

Generally, marital functioning over the 1-year period remained stable in the close relationships. When asked what was critical to maintaining a good relationship, partners described the maintenance of each other's autonomy, the use of empathy in responding to each other, and open communication. Complementary, synchronized functioning and collaboration were essential (Cannon 1997).

Written Surveys

Survey results enabled a closer, inside view of these relationships. How do couples cope with progressive losses due to A1AD? Even as uncontrollable losses occur in lung function, physical abilities, and social involvement, couples in good marriages stated that they had gained more than they had lost, finding new activities to do together and a deeper intimacy within their relationship. Many of the partners discovered new opportunities to learn and to be involved with others who face similar challenges. Life goals were revised, with a greater focus on "living each day" by refocusing on the positive and the important. Strategies for accepting the illness, as well as reliance on faith to endure its burdens, were offered as good ways to cope with losses. Some felt that the ability to walk away from some problems was the best way to deal with them (Cannon 1997).

When well spouses were asked, "What do you do to make your partner feel better?" they stated that they gave love, time, encouragement, and help when needed. They worked to help their spouses maintain self-esteem and physical health. When the spouses with A1AD answered the same question, they stated that they worked hard to adapt to illness, stay independent, enjoy life, express gratitude, and maintain a positive attitude. The ill spouses encouraged the autonomy of their well spouses, supported their goals, shared love, and planned time to be together (Cannon 1997).

Comparisons of Functioning and Coping Between More and Less Satisfying Marriages

Sample Description

In addition to the focus group couples, 182 partners in A1AD-affected marriages throughout the world completed mailed surveys containing well-established measures of partner and marital characteristics, functioning, coping, and outcomes of well-being. In order to describe the ways the most satisfying marriages manage the breathlessness and progressive losses due to A1AD, the couples were clustered into two groups using the sum and difference scores on the Dyadic Adjustment Scale (Spanier 1976) and a rating scale for perceived marital happiness. The two clusters were similar in the distribution of sex, mean age, percent having had transplants, and percent taking Prolastin. Statistically significant differences in mean number of years of education, income range, percent employed, and average ages since symptom onset and diagnosis were found, with those in less satisfying marriages scoring lower in each parameter.

Marital Functioning

When marital functioning of patients and spouses in more satisfying marriages was compared with functioning of partners in less satisfying marriages using the Family Assessment Measure III, Dyadic Relationship Scale (Skinner 1984), significant differences in affective functioning, affective involvement, and control were found. In other words, the more satisfied couples viewed their marriages as sources of security, concern, empathy, and nurturing that fostered the autonomy of each partner. Marriage was experienced as a safe place, where a wide range of feelings could be expressed and where predictable, but flexible, patterns of interpersonal influence existed. The flexibility allowed shifts in functioning to meet changing demands (Cannon 1997).

Coping Strategies

To further study the strategies used in more satisfying marriages to cope with the stress of A1AD, the Brief COPE measure (Carver 1994) and relationship-focused strategy scales (Coyne 1991, O'Brien 1991) were applied. Within mutually satisfying marriages, patients used the following strategies to deal with stress significantly more than their well spouses:

1. active coping—exerting efforts to remove or circumvent stressors
2. distraction—refocusing and not dwelling on stressful situations

3. behavioral disengagement—giving up behaviors to cope with stress
4. alcohol and/or drug use
5. venting—expressing unpleasant or negative feelings

The strategies of active coping and distraction may be helpful to patients in controlling stress, while the well spouses in satisfying marriages may have less need to use avoidance strategies. In these marriages, well spouses used the relationship-focused strategy of empathic responding significantly more than their ill partners (Cannon 1997).

In contrast, less satisfying marriages were characterized by the significantly higher use of emotional venting and behavioral disengagement by well spouses (compared with well spouses in more satisfying marriages). A higher use of distraction and protective buffering (hiding problems and feelings from each other) was found in both less satisfied partners. Within these marriages, well spouses reported a higher use of alcohol and drugs than their ill partners, although under-reporting is suspected. These findings suggest that a distance exists between partners, leaving little opportunity for communication and the sharing of feelings, thus preventing the type of collaboration needed to deal with the invasiveness of symptoms (Cannon 1997).

Selected Outcomes

Patients in more satisfying marriages reported significantly less frequent symptoms of depression than patients in less satisfying marriages, as measured on the CES-D scale (Radloff 1977). Partners in more satisfying marriages perceived a significantly higher competence in dealing with their feelings than partners in less satisfying marriages. In contrast, partners in less satisfying marriages reported increased severity of stress caused by the wheezing, coughing, and infections that accompany A1AD (Cannon 1997, 1999).

Conclusions

Identifying the ways that partners in satisfying marriages manage and adapt as A1AD emphysema advances has provided suggestions to the multidisciplinary team for helping couples with less experience with the illness and greater difficulties in managing the illness-marital trajectory. So what has been learned about living with the advancing breathlessness and progressive losses of A1AD in the context of marriage?

1. The illness provides a unique opportunity to exhibit love and closeness—to put the marriage to work.
2. Longer experiences with managing A1AD provide a perspective that allows the past to inform the present and prepare for the future. With

advancing symptoms, limitations increase and the outside world becomes more threatening.

3. Over time, satisfying marriages remain stable. Friendship and intimacy take on new meanings as long as the marriage remains a safe place to express feelings. Flexible, yet predictable, patterns of interpersonal functioning allow couples to remain, or become, synchronous in meeting their needs.

4. Overprotectiveness is not healthy for either spouse. Shielding each other from information may lead to anger and failure to control the situation, resulting in negative outcomes for both partners.

5. Satisfying marriages function as sources of nurturing, while less satisfying marriages may actually become the sources of stress.

References

Bradbury, TN and FD Fincham. 1989. Behavior and satisfaction in marriage: prospective mediating processes. *Rev Personality Social Psych.* 10:119-143.

Brantly, ML, LD Paul, BH Miller, RT Falk, M Wu, and RG Crystal. 1988. Clinical features and history of the destructive lung disease associated with alpha 1-antitrypsin deficiency of adults with pulmonary symptoms. *Am Rev Resp Dis.* 138:327-336.

Burr, WR, WR Klein et al. 1994. *Reexamining Family Stress.* Thousand Oaks, CA: Sage.

Cannon, CA. 1997. *Marital Stress and Coping in Alpha 1-Antitrypsin Deficiency.* Ann Arbor, MI: UMI Dissertation Services.

———. 1998. Themes of marital stress and coping in alpha 1. *A1AD Q Rev.* 2(1):3-5.

———. 1999. Severity and sources of stress in alpha 1-antitrypsin deficiency. Poster presented at A1AD Investigators Conference, San Diego, CA (Apr 24).

Carver, CS. 1994. Brief COPE Measure.

Coyne, JC and DA Smith. 1991. Couples coping with a myocardial infarction: a contextual perspective on wives' distress. *J Personality Social Psych.* 61(3):404-412.

Larrson, C. 1978. Natural history and life expectancy in severe alpha 1-antitrypsin deficiency, PiZ. *Acta Medicus Scandinavia.* 204:345-351.

Lazarus, R and S Folkman. 1984. *Stress, Appraisal, and Coping.* New York: Springer.

O'Brien, T and A DeLongis. 1991. *A three-function model of coping: emotion-focused, problem-focused, and relationship-focused.* Paper presented at the Annual Meeting of the American Psychological Association. San Francisco, CA.

Radloff, LS. 1977. The CES-D scale: a self-report depression scale for research in the general population. *App Psych Measurement.* 1:385-401.

Skinner, HA, PD Steinhauer, and J Santa-Barbara. 1984. *Family Assessment Measure.* New York: Multi-Health Systems.

Spanier, GB. 1976. Measuring dyadic adjustment: new scales for assessing the quality of marriage and similar dyads. *J Marriage Family.* 38:15-28.

Steinhauer, PD, J Santa-Barbara, and HA Skinner. 1984. The process model of family functioning. *Can J Psych.* 29:77-88.

Stoller, JK, P Smith, P Yang, and J Spray. 1994. Physical and social impact of alpha 1-antitrypsin deficiency: results of a survey. *Cleveland Clinic J Med.* Nov-Dec: 461-467.

Strauss, A and J Corbin. 1990. *Basics of Qualitative Research.* Newbury Park, CA: Sage.

Thibaut, JW and HH Kelley. 1959. *The Social Psychology of Groups.* New York: John Wiley.

Whitchurch, GG and LL Constantine. 1993. Systems theory. In *Sourcebook of Family Theories and Methods*, eds. G Boss, WJ Doherty, R LaRossa, WR Schumm, and SK Steinmetz, 325-352. New York: Plenum Press.

9

We're More Than a Chart:
Treating the Whole Person

Julie Swanson

The author is past president of Alpha 1 Association (www.alpha1.org). Here she recounts her own experiences and views as a person with alpha 1-antitrypsin deficiency (A1AD) and how her son's cystic fibrosis affected her approach to own her illness.

In October 1987, I went to my family doctor with a complaint of bronchitis. An x-ray was taken that showed some infiltration in the right middle lobe, and I was treated with antibiotics over the course of several months. I had some improvement, but the cough still hung on. Five months later, I had another x-ray taken that showed even more infiltration than did the previous film in October. I was referred to a pulmonary specialist who asked an array of questions and ran several tests, including a sweat test for cystic fibrosis and a test for A1AD. The test results came back positive for A1AD. Complete pulmonary function testing was done that showed an FEV_1 of 1.13, which was only 39% of predicted. What a shock!

My doctor informed me that there was a new replacement therapy starting to hit the market, but a good amount of data was not available yet. In addition, other factors had to be considered, such as the very high cost of the drug and the risk of contracting hepatitis or AIDS, which was on the rise and tragically affecting the hemophilia community. But the biggest fear I had was that our insurance company might cancel us if I chose to go on the replacement therapy. It had been so hard to get coverage in the first place because of our son having cystic fibrosis (CF). I just could not take a chance of losing his coverage, and we decided that the risk was too great at that time.

For the next 2 years I watched as my lung function dropped. My FEV_1 was down to .64, which was 20% of predicted. I had no choice but to try the replacement therapy, Prolastin. In May 1990, I received my first dose of the drug, and I have remained stable ever since. In hindsight, I sure wish I had gotten on it sooner. I do believe, though, that it is not just one method but a combination of approaches that leads me to do so well.

Proactive Approaches

Positive Attitude

By the time I was diagnosed with A1AD, I had already developed a very proactive approach to chronic illness because of my experience with our son's CF. Our family had decided that no matter how short Jacob's life was to be, we would not treat him as a sick child. We were not going to put him in a bubble. Whatever he wanted to try, we would let him try, and we have kept him very active in sports and exercise. Jacob just celebrated his 14th birthday, a birthday we thought we would never see. He does very well and is such a well-adjusted, positive kid. I remember once, when he was about 10 years old, him talking on the phone to one of my friends and telling her that he wanted to bungee jump. She said, "Aren't you scared?" He simply replied, "No, life is too short to be scared." What a great outlook he has.

Such a positive attitude is not only for patients, though. Physicians must have it, too. For the first couple of years after my diagnosis, I so badly wanted my doctor to give me the answer to the question, "How long do I have?" I thought he should know that, and I wanted to know. I would look up my FEV_1 in medical books and come back to him and say, "The book says that I have less than 5 years to live. Is this true?" He would explain that there are so many variables that there is no way of predicting. On the drive home, I would be thinking, "Darn! He squirmed out of it again." I just knew he had to know. After all, he is a doctor. Well, here I am, 11 years later. I did manage to get over that obsession and I do believe now that there really are many variables that make a difference in the course of a disease. I think that the biggest variable is a positive attitude. In looking back, I am glad that he never tried to give me an answer to my question because it might have made things worse. My doctor admits that he was very worried during those first couple of years because my lung function was dropping so quickly. But he, too, kept a positive attitude and took a lot of time answering my questions. If he did not have the answer, he took the time to find out and get back to me.

Education

When I was diagnosed, I used the same approach for myself that I used with my son. I was not going to put myself in a bubble. Instead, I would educate myself about the disease and do what I needed to do to stay healthy. At the time I was diagnosed, it was hard to find any information on A1AD and impossible to find something in layman's terms. Education is an important factor in doing well. In my experience as an alpha and in talking to a lot of alphas, the more educated we are about the disease, the better we do. Education also promotes a good attitude because we do not have a fear of the unknown. I feel it is important for physicians to encourage patients to be proactive and to learn about their disease. Physicians should link their patients up with organizations like the Alpha 1 Association, whose mission includes education and which offers a lot of wonderful information. I have been very lucky that I have a doctor who let me know that I was his first and only A1AD patient at the time. He told me that he did not have a lot of knowledge about treating A1AD, so we would be learning together. We have a partnership in controlling my disease. I feel very comfortable bringing him new information that I come across or relaying ideas that have worked for other alphas. Good two-way communication between physician and patient is critical in a successful partnership and in controlling a chronic illness.

Support of Others With A1AD

Although I had a good partnership with my doctor and great support from my family, something was still missing—the support of people who truly knew what I was feeling, people who had already walked the path I was now on. I needed someone who could help lead me through the emotions encountered by the diagnosis of A1AD. I needed someone I could share fears, concerns, and dreams with. Unfortunately, at the time I was diagnosed, there was no A1AD association to which to turn. Now there is. Alpha 1 Association supports not only alphas but physicians as well, and it is an organization that physicians should rely on heavily. It became very important to me to get involved with the Alpha 1 Association. I did not want other alphas to go through what I did—having no one to compare notes with, having no good information that I could understand, and feeling scared and alone even though I had wonderful support from my family. My family had enough stress from coping with our son's illness; I did not want to add to it.

The Alpha 1 Association has a successful Family and Peer Support Program, which has been received very well. A newly diagnosed alpha is carefully matched with a peer counselor, another alpha with a similar situation who has gone through training and is willing to share his or her experiences. On average, the Association receives 185 calls and e-mails each day and the numbers continually grow. Physicians can help the Alpha 1 Association meet its demands by becoming a member and help patients by encouraging them to get support.

Impact on Family

What is the impact of chronic illness on a family? It affects every member differently. There is a lot of stress from many angles. The person with the disease may feel guilty and feel as though he or she is a burden. The spouse feels helpless and scared, not wanting the other to die first. The kids also feel helpless and scared. They see the trouble the ill person has when playing with them. When our son was diagnosed with CF, I remember being told that it would either make our marriage stronger or lead to a divorce. I was one of the lucky ones. It made our marriage stronger. In our family, I do not think we dwell on it much, unless Jacob is or I am sick. We realize time is too short. Whether people have a chronic illness or not, they do not know when it's going to be their time. The illness has given us the gift of realizing that.

What major life changes occur as the disease progresses? Often, the patient has to retire at an early age. If it is the husband who is ill, he does not feel like he is able to provide for his family, be the breadwinner, or be the strong figure of the household. The wife has to take over the heavier chores. Now he sees himself as weak, failing, and a burden. If it is a woman who has the chronic illness, she feels the same low self-esteem. She feels that she is failing because she cannot keep up with the family like she used to. She is unable to contribute to the family income. She is frustrated at not being able to play with the kids and keep up with normal daily activities. Chores get switched around to compensate.

Families dealing with chronic illness are faced with planning days carefully and prioritizing activities. The energy level of the ill person changes daily. There are days that I cannot walk from one room to another. Those days I refer to as my "humbling days" because it makes me realize how lucky I am that I usually do so well. Another problem that A1AD patients have to deal with is that many of us do not look sick. Even family members occasionally forget that we do have our limitations. We are faced with a lot of stress, stress from the Prolastin shortage, and stress from the financial impact of the disease. We are conscious of what a change in employment can mean. Will the new job have good health care benefits? Am I or my spouse going to get laid off from our jobs because of the medical claims we file?

What Patients Need From Their Physicians

We need to feel that we are more than just a chart. We need encouragement to not give up, especially when we are struggling during our illness. We need to know that our physicians are truly committed to the partnership. We need to know that they are being up front with us.

We need pulmonary rehab, so we can learn how to watch for warning signs while we are exercising and so we have the motivation needed to increase our limits. Physicians need to reinforce the fact that any exercise is better then none at all. That if we start out with just two minutes of exercise a day and increase it in small increments, we will see improvements in our daily lives. Physicians should take the time to explain the importance of exercise, of letting our muscles do the work instead of our lungs.

Physicians need to review the way that they give oxygen saturation tests. Just having a patient walk down the hall a few times does not give a correct assessment. I went to my doctor and told him that I was having problems while exercising and that maybe we should check into prescribing oxygen with exercise. So, down the hall we went and my saturation stayed up there pretty well. I said, "OK, I guess I don't need it. It is just part of the disease and I'll have to live with it." When I went back in for my next check-up, though, I mentioned it again. "It sure seems like I could use oxygen when I'm exercising." Back out in the hall we went and I did fine again, but this time I suggested that we try the stairs. We went up one flight of stairs and I dropped to 87% on my saturation. We went back to the office and he wrote a prescription for oxygen. Several people have had the same experience that I had with the saturation test and I told them my story. Sure enough, when they were re-tested using the stairs, their doctors ended up prescribing oxygen with exercise. I am also hearing from more and more alphas that when sleep studies were done to assess their oxygen needs at night, the results showed that they should be on oxygen during sleep. Physicians must trust that we patients know our own bodies better than others can.

We need physicians to stress the importance of educating the family members on the genetic aspect of A1AD. I hear many stories of how a family member was diagnosed, but no information was passed on or testing done on the family members. Then, years later, problems show up. No one told them what symptoms to watch for or that they must not to smoke. It is so sad when that happens. Damage could possibly have been prevented if they had only known.

What can physicians do to make patients' lives a little easier? Make it possible for chronically ill patients to communicate with them directly or get in to see them as needed. There is nothing worse for patients than to know that they are coming down with something but not be able to get past a physician's "nurse from hell." Physicians need to educate patients on what signs to look for that indicate an onset of an illness. Physicians should have patients contact them at the first symptom and not wait until it develops into a full cold or bronchitis. Physicians should start treating patients at the very onset of an illness.

What do patients not want? We do not want to feel that physicians are trying to rush through appointments and not really listening to us.

What are our biggest obstacles and how best can physicians help? For many patients, health care coverage is one of our biggest obstacles. HMOs are on the increase and, frankly, they do not work for people with chronic illness. I am presently going through a change with our health insurance. I picked my primary doctor as required because, of course, my family doctor was not on their list. I called to make an appointment and was told that the first available appointment was in 2 months. I explained to them that my son and I needed to have prescriptions filled and we needed referrals to our specialists. Well, those could not be done until we meet with the primary doctor but, no, we could not get in sooner. In the meantime, I have had to give up my pulmonary rehab program because I could not get in to my doctor to get it approved under the new insurance. This type of situation is so aggravating and stressful, and it wears on us. Patients have enough to worry about without adding the nightmare of insurance. We need physicians' help in trying to correct this situation. They should voice their concerns regarding health care issues to Congress. Let medical associations know that they want these issues addressed for the benefit of their patients; voice their concerns about how HMO patients have to jump though hoops just to be able to get an appointment with their specialists.

Each patient is an individual; there is no one blueprint to follow in treating one of us. The Alpha 1 Association has information for patients, for family members, and for physicians. Physicians should use this resource.

It is obvious to me that many professionals involved with A1AD are concerned and caring, with a thirst for new knowledge in the treatment of chronic illnesses. I applaud their efforts and encourage them to continue to come together to further their commitment to the care of the chronically ill.

10

Smoking Cessation

Kevin R. Cooper, MD

Cigarette consumption in the United States has been declining since it reached a per capita peak in 1964. The highest smoking rates by birth cohort (US DHHS 1991) were seen in men born between 1911 and 1930 (66% were daily smokers when they were age 20-40) and women born between 1931 and 1940 (44% daily smokers at age 20-40). As smokers age, some die of smoking-related diseases, and many others quit smoking, so that by age 70, only 17% of the 1911-1920 male birth cohort were still smoking. People born more recently have smoked less. For example, smoking peaked at about 30% for both sexes born between 1960 and 1970, and has already begun to decline for this age cohort. In 1994, the prevalence of current smoking by Americans over age 65 was 13.2% of men and 11.1% of women (Husten 1997). Among men over age 65, 81.5% of those who had ever smoked had quit, compared with 70.7% of women. Smoking rates were higher and quit ratios were lower for blacks than for whites. Despite a downward trend in the *percentage* of adults over 65 who are smokers, the *number* is growing, totaling 3.7 million in 1994.

Beginning in the 1880s, many more men than women smoked, leading to a much greater prevalence of smoking-related diseases among men. The male predominance at all ages is now disappearing. Among 12th graders, 19% described themselves as frequent smokers in 1997 (US DHHS 1998). The rate is actually slightly greatly for white girls than white boys, while black and Hispanic girls smoke less than their male counterparts.

About 20% of daily smokers develop chronic obstructive lung disease (COPD). By the time COPD reaches an advanced stage, most smokers know that cigarette smoking has caused the illness. A few continue to maintain that an occupational exposure or ambient air pollution is really to blame, but the connection between smoking and emphysema is certainly common knowledge. Family members have often been trying for years to persuade the patient to quit. This situation illustrates the best definition of addiction, ie, using a substance to provide pleasure despite the knowledge that it has harmful or even fatal consequences. A smoker who has already reached such a stage of debility that he gets dyspneic walking across the room and has given up favorite activities like golf, hunting, or even mowing the lawn has long ago made the choice that he prefers the pleasure of cigarettes to the health benefits of quitting. What can a health care provider do at this late stage to change this smoker's mind?

The first step in getting patients to reconsider is to convince them that the decision to continue smoking is based on faulty information. Most smokers with advanced disease began smoking before tobacco's health effects were widely accepted, and they may still underestimate both the risks of smoking and the benefits of quitting. They easily adopt the idea that "it's too late now for quitting to do any good." Each patient must be convinced that quitting smoking, even when COPD is at an advanced stage, increases both lifespan and the quality of life. The 1990 Surgeon General's Report emphasizes that "it is never too late to quit smoking," and 3 out of 4 people over age 65 who have ever smoked have already quit (Husten 1997).

Effect on Survival

The earlier a person quits smoking, the greater the survival benefit. Quitting before age 50 reduces the risk of dying before age 65 by 50%, but quitting between ages 60 and 64 reduces the risk of dying in the next 15 years by only 10% (US DHHS 1990, Cox 1993). The benefit of quitting is somewhat underestimated by these numbers because many people over age 60 quit smoking after learning that they have a potentially fatal smoking-induced disease.

The most immediate benefit of quitting is a reduction in the risk of death due to arteriosclerosis, the disease that kills more American smokers than any other. The 5% to 10% carboxyhemoglobin level common among smokers increases both symptomatic and silent episodes of cardiac ischemia, increasing the risk of infarction, arythmia, and sudden death. After smoking cessation, the carbon monoxide level decreases to normal within about 12 hours, reducing the risk of death. After 1 year of smoke-free living, the risk of dying of myocardial infarction has declined by 50%, and continues to decline further with time. The risk of stroke also drops immediately, and then steadily diminishes until it approaches the risk of a never-smoker by 10 years after quitting. The fear of a paralyzing stroke, leading to dependence on family or other caregivers for activities of daily living, can sometimes be a more effective motivation for quitting than the fear of sudden death.

The likelihood of developing cancer is also reduced by smoking cessation, but much more slowly. Five years after smoking cessation, the risk of lung cancer has declined by about 25% compared with continuing smokers, and there follows a gradual decline over the next 25 years, approaching but not equaling the risk of never-smokers. Survival in other cancers shows a similar pattern. Although a reduced cancer risk may always be perceived as a benefit, it does not carry the same impact for an older patient with advanced COPD as it does for a younger, healthier smoker.

COPD worsens at a faster rate among people who continue smoking than among those who quit. After quitting smoking, the loss of pulmonary function parallels the normal rate of decline in nonsmokers, whereas decline is much faster in continuing smokers (Speizer 1979). The message that emphysema gets worse with time even among those who quit smoking is not good news for patients, but quitting maximizes survival and can improve respiratory symptoms and health-related quality of life even though pulmonary function does not improve.

Quitting is beneficial to many areas of the human body. Current smokers have a 1.5-2.0 relative risk of hip fracture compared with former and never-smokers (LaCroix 1992). About 220,000 older Americans suffer hip fracture each year and 10% die from complications. Mobility is impaired for survivors and 50% of them are discharged from the hospital to a nursing home.

A smoker who quits will almost always add some life expectancy. The amount varies according to individual circumstances, but the average 65-year-old smoker has 4 years less life remaining than people who have never smoked, and quitting at age 65 restores 2 of those 4 years (Sachs 1986). Smokers who are older or sicker can expect to add less lifespan, but even a gain of a month may be very important when one's remaining time is short.

Positive Effects on Quality of Life

Smokers with advanced COPD have usually considered the reduced longevity of smokers but continue to smoke anyway, because the increased longevity is an abstract statistical benefit, while the pleasure of cigarettes is real and immediate. Emphasizing the benefits of smoking cessation on the quality of life may be more persuasive. Health-related quality of life improves after smoking cessation (Tillman 1997, Hirdes 1994), especially with regard to respiratory symptoms. However, smokers also fear negative effects on quality of life, and counselors must be open to discuss both aspects.

Daily cough and sputum usually abate completely after smoking cessation in smokers with simple chronic bronchitis (without obstructive lung disease), but in smokers with advanced COPD the effect of smoking cessation on cough and sputum is more variable. All smokers should be aware that cough and sputum often get worse during the first month after quitting. Most can accept this as a period during which the lungs "clean out" the tar that they have inhaled over the years (in fact, it is because some components of smoke inflame the airways but others suppress cough). During subsequent months, inflammation subsides and cough and sputum diminish, but often not completely. Continued treatment with bronchodilators, anti-inflammatory agents, and sometimes mucolytics and antibiotics often improve these symptoms.

For some patients, avoidance of disability may be a more potent motivator than prolonging life. Personal risk factors for disabling diseases should be explained to smokers to make the concern more personal and less

75

abstract. Emphasizing the additive effect of concomitant risk factors for arteriosclerosis, such as hypertension and diabetes, can make avoiding a stroke by smoking cessation a more urgent concern. Quitting smoking usually improves the ability to exercise without pain for patients with intermittent claudication, and reduces the chance that amputation will be necessary.

Many co-existing diseases are accelerated or worsened by smoking, and the associated disability may be a powerful motivator. Peptic ulcer disease and gastroesophageal reflux are helped by smoking cessation. A patient with macular degeneration may fear blindness enough to stop smoking when he learns that smokers with over 40 "pack-years" have 5 times the risk of advanced degenerative retinal changes (Delcourt 1998). A woman with osteoporosis may fear the hip fracture and nursing home enough to quit smoking. A diabetic with nephropathy should be told that progression to end-stage renal disease and dialysis is twice as fast for smokers as for nonsmokers (Orth 1997). A patient with cataracts who fears surgery may quit smoking when he learns that smoking accelerates the progression of cataracts.

Negative Effects on Quality of Life

When health and vigor are slipping away in smokers with advanced COPD, they are likely to cling to remaining sources of solace and pleasure. Cigarettes are often one of life's few remaining pleasures. While health care providers are frustrated by the patient's seeming delusion that it is in his best interest to keep smoking, what counselors sometimes fail to appreciate is the power of nicotine to provide pleasure. By the time a smoker has COPD, he has usually been enjoying the effects of nicotine for 30-50 years. Nicotine is a drug that can stimulate the brain's dopaminergic-mesolimbic system, creating sensations of reward and pleasure, or the locus ceruleus, enhancing vigilance and alertness, depending on the smoker's desire at a given moment.

Smokers perform better on tests of memory and physical agility when allowed to smoke ad lib, and the self-administration of nicotine can create a feeling of being in control, just when the smoker is losing control over daily activities because of the limitations imposed by COPD. Each puff gives a dose of nicotine, and the average smoker self-administers 200 puffs per day. Since nicotine is so effective at improving the way smokers feel about life experiences, the prospect of giving it up can seem like a huge loss of ability to cope with everyday stress. Smokers even help themselves deal with the symptoms and limitations of COPD by using cigarettes. The satisfaction provided by nicotine is so powerful that some ex-smokers have equated quitting to losing an old friend or a lover.

Studies of Older Smokers

A survey of older smokers' characteristics and attitudes was conducted in 1988 (Rimer 1990). Among respondents aged 50-74, 11% were smokers, 47% former smokers, and 42% never-smokers. Smokers had been smoking for an average of 46 years. Although more men than women had been smokers at some time in their lives, 87% of the men who had ever smoked had quit, compared with only 69% of the women. The higher quit rates for men than for women is consistent with results of other studies. Twenty-nine percent of current smokers were married to smokers, compared with only 10% of former smokers. This raises two important points: (1) cessation success rates for smokers married to smokers is much higher when both spouses attempt quitting together, and (2) the social support system of smokers is likely to include smokers. When older smokers give up nicotine, they may also face a major change in, or even the loss of, long established supportive relationships with friends and family.

In the survey, smokers had much higher rates of COPD and respiratory symptoms than ex- and never-smokers, and twice as many described their present health as poor. Even so, smokers were less likely to have seen a doctor in the last year and less likely to have had health screening tests such as mammograms, stool tests for occult blood, and blood pressure checks. As a group, smokers were underserved by health care providers, even after adjustments for socioeconomic status and educational achievement.

The survey showed a clear need for education about health effects. Forty-seven percent of current smokers did not believe that quitting smoking could improve their health, and 45% did not believe that continued smoking would cause them harm. These misperceptions are a major impediment to smoking cessation, and health care providers need to work with patients to correct them. Stratifying responses by age showed that the older the smoker, the less likely he or she was to believe that cessation was worthwhile. A study by Clark, Rakowski et al (1997) found that among smokers over age 50, those who had a realistic understanding of the health consequences of smoking and believed that smoking is addictive were more likely to quit.

Cigarette consumption is also an important factor. Coambs, Li, and Kozlowski (1992) found that among smokers under age 45, the lighter smokers were more likely to quit, but for those 45 and older, the heavier smokers had a higher cessation rate. They concede that heavier smokers are generally more addicted, but speculate that the light smoking group over age 45 includes strongly addicted smokers who were formerly heavy smokers that have cut down, rather than quit, after experiencing negative health effects.

The best smoking cessation success rate is among patients who have recently had a critical event related to the heart. Quit rates above 50% are reported after myocardial infarction or even coronary angiography without infarction (Ockene 1992). A diagnosis of COPD or cancer may also lead to a decision to quit smoking, but less often.

Older smokers who are asked about quitting are worried that they will experience cravings (68%), get irritable or anxious (52%), gain weight (47%), and feel bored (42%) and only 39% said that their physicians had recommended quitting in the last year (Orleans 1991). Even though it has been 10 years since this survey was conducted, and many of these older smokers did not have COPD, it seems clear that physicians and other health care providers are missing opportunities to tell smokers to quit and to point out the benefits of quitting.

Fisher and Hill (1990) emphasize that social isolation is an important barrier to smoking cessation. The shorter male lifespan as well as women's lower success rate at smoking cessation means that there are many widows who live alone and smoke. Because of their feeling of loss and lone survivorship, it may seem less worthwhile to them to undertake a difficult change in lifestyle with the goal of adding more years of life.

Smoking and Depression

The interaction of smoking and depression is complex. Judging by questionnaires, smokers are more depressed than nonsmokers, and a history of major depression is common in those seeking smoking cessation services. Even so, nicotine use can help smokers deal with depressive symptoms. Clearly, many smokers experience a sense of achievement and a boost in self-esteem after quitting, but smokers who have a history of major depression are at an increased risk of another major depression after quitting smoking (Covey 1998). Even among highly addicted smokers who have not had major depression, a sense of loss often accompanies giving up cigarettes, sometimes as deep as the loss of a spouse. Smoking is different from other losses, however, because the smoker can always decide to resurrect the pleasure and companionship that was lost (Ferguson 1987, Cooper 1997). Senses of loss and achievement are felt simultaneously, and the net effect on each smoker varies greatly.

Although bupropion is an antidepressant, its effectiveness as a smoking cessation adjunct does not depend on its antidepressant action, since it is also effective in smokers who are not depressed. Other antidepressants are of minimal or no benefit in smoking cessation.

Approach to Smoking Cessation

The success rate for quitting smoking among people over age 65 is comparable to success rates among younger adults. Orleans et al (1994) reported a 6-month success rate of 28% for older smokers trying to quit with the help of the nicotine patch. Dale et al (1997) found a 25% success rate 6 months after a consultation at Mayo Clinic's Nicotine Dependence Center. Even a single visit with a physician who advises smoking cessation, followed up by a contact in 6 months, yielded a 14% quit rate compared with a 9% quit rate among controls (Vetter 1990). Yet health care providers often do not even tell their smoking patients to quit.

A smoker becomes an ex-smoker by a sequence of changes described by Prochaska et al (1992). Precontemplation is a stage of happily enjoying the benefits of nicotine, followed by contemplation of quitting. The smoker makes preparation, and eventually takes action, tries to quit, and is either successful, entering a maintenance stage, or relapses and goes back to the precontemplation stage. What happens at the time of relapse is crucial. The smoker may believe that this failure means that the task is impossible and that he will always fail. The counselor should praise abstinence of any duration as a foundation to build on for greater success on the next attempt. Since there are more ex-smokers than current smokers in the United States, quitting is not only possible, it is the usual conclusion to a smoking habit. At each step in this sequence of psychological stages, the counselor should help the patient move to the next stage and not try to skip stages. Hopefully, after some number of attempts, a durable abstinence is achieved and the patient is an ex-smoker. It is important to approach patients at a "teachable moment," when they are more open to considering a change in lifestyle because of recent life events. For example, smoking cessation counseling that is begun in the hospital has a higher rate of success than efforts initiated as an outpatient (Dale 1997).

Health care providers do not need extensive training in smoking cessation techniques. The National Institutes of Health has proven that a simple approach of "4 A's" is effective: *ask* all patients if they smoke, *advise* them to quit, *assist* them in the effort, and *arrange* follow-up for this problem. Assisting may include counseling, providing self-help materials, and recommending nicotine replacement or bupropion. Follow-up may consist of continued counseling during subsequent visits, referral to an organized smoking cessation program, or telephone contacts during the cessation effort.

It is more effective to involve each patient in planning his or her own cessation effort than to use the same approach for everyone. There are many different options to try: groups, hypnosis, relaxation techniques, books, step-by-step plans on videotape, etc. While nicotine replacement and bupropion increase the success rate when added to a cessation effort, they are not stand-alone approaches that will ensure that someone quits. The health care provider must help the patient progress to the contemplation stage, construct an action plan in partnership with the patient, and then agree on a quit date.

Smoking Reduction

Quitting completely is best, but a substantial reduction in cigarette consumption may also yield important benefits. The risk of lung cancer increases linearly in proportion to the number of cigarettes smoked in a lifetime. The risk of other diseases is more difficult to define statistically but probably follows a similar dose/response relationship. Cutting down from 30 to 10 cigarettes a day, therefore, may reduce the health risk by as much as 60%, but the actual benefit for each individual is variable because of changes in the way that each cigarette is smoked while cutting down. Smokers who are cutting down tend to take more and deeper puffs from each cigarette, especially when smoking fewer than 10 cigarettes a day.

The psychological benefit of cutting down can be substantial, especially when the health care provider reacts to this news with congratulations for partial success, rather than negativity: "So why don't you cut out the other 10?" Patients who have plateaued at a fraction of their former cigarette use should be supported against backsliding and encouraged to cut a little more when the time is right.

Risk Reduction Without Cessation

The importance of diet is often overlooked. Smokers whose diet (with or without supplements) resulted in high levels of alpha-tocopherol had a 20% lower risk of lung cancer (Woodson 1999). Diets resulting in high serum levels of beta carotene also reduce lung cancer risk (Menkes 1986), but simply adding a beta carotene supplement does not help. The effect of diet on progression of COPD is unknown, but, theoretically, dietary antioxidants may reduce the risk of COPD and other smoking-related diseases as well. Adding foods rich in vitamins A and E (fruits, vegetables, and whole grains) may represent a helpful strategy for all smokers, especially those who do not stop smoking. While the exact benefit of vitamin E supplements is still under study, current data warrant advising smokers to take a supplement. Regular exercise has not been shown to improve survival, but reduces hospitalizations and improves performance status and quality of life.

Summary

Cigarette smoking is the cause of over 90% of COPD but is ultimately a modifiable behavior. Health care providers should emphasize the following points.

1. One is never too old to benefit from quitting smoking.
2. Significant improvements in both quantity and quality of life can be expected.

3. Past failed attempts do not predict future failure. In fact, the average ex-smoker has tried to quit 5 times before the final successful attempt.
4. Nicotine withdrawal can be curtailed by nicotine replacement therapy.
5. Bupropion may help diminish the desire to smoke and should be considered.

References

Clark, MA, W Rakowski, FJ Kviz, and JW Hogan. 1997. Age and stage of readiness for smoking cessation. *J Gerontol B Psychol Sci Soc Sci.* 52(4):S122-221.

Coambs, RB, S Li, and LT Kozlowski. 1992. Age interacts with heaviness of smoking in predicting success in cessation of smoking. *Am J Epidem.* 135:240-246.

Cooper, KR. 1997. Smoking cessation. In *A Practical Approach to Pulmonary Medicine*, eds. RH Goldstein, JJ O'Connell, and JB Karlinsky, 503-511. Philadelphia, PA: Lippincott-Raven.

Covey, LS, AH Glassman, and F Stetner. 1998. Cigarette smoking and major depression. *J Addict Dis.* 17(1):35-46.

Cox, JL. 1993. Smoking cessation in the elderly patient. *Clinics in Chest Med.* 14(3):423-428.

Dale, LC, DA Olsen, CA Patten et al. 1997. Predictors of smoking cessation among elderly smokers treated for nicotine dependence. *Tob Control.* 6(3):181-187.

Delcourt, C, JL Diaz, A Ponton-Sanchez, and L Papoz. 1998. Smoking and age-related macular degeneration: the POLA study. *Arch Ophthalmol.* 116:1031-1035.

Ferguson, T. 1987. *The No-nag, No-guilt, Do-it-your own-way Guide to Quitting Smoking.* 17-27. New York: Ballantine.

Fisher, EB and RD Hill. 1990. Perspectives on older smokers. *Chest.* 97(3):517-518.

Hirdes, JP and CJ Maxwell. 1994. Smoking cessation and quality of life outcomes among older adults in the Campbell's survey on well-being. *Can J Pub Hlth.* 85:99-102.

Husten, CG, DM Shelton, JH Chrismon et al. 1997. Cigarette smoking and smoking cessation among older adults: United States, 1965-94. *Tob Control.* 6(3):175-180.

LaCroix, AZ and GS Omenn. 1992. Older adults and smoking. *Clinics in Ger Med.* 8(1):69-87.

Menkes, MS, GW Comstock, JP Vuilleumier et al. 1986. Serum beta-carotene, vitamins A and E, selenium, and the risk of lung cancer. *New Eng J Med.* 315:1250-1254.

Ockene, J, JL Kristeller, R Goldberg et al. 1992. Smoking cessation and severity of disease: the coronary artery smoking intervention study. *Hlth Psych.* 11(2):119-126.

Orleans, CT, BK Rimer, S Cristinzio et al. 1991. A national survey of older smokers: treatment needs of a growing population. *Hlth Psych.* 10(5):343-351.

Orleans, CT, N Resch, E Noll et al. 1994. Use of transdermal nicotine in a state level prescription plan for the elderly: a first look at 'real-world patch users.' *JAMA.* 271:601-607.

Orth, SR, E Ritz, and RW Schrier. 1997. The renal risks of smoking. *Kidney Int.* 51:1669-1677.

Prochaska, JO, CC DiClemente, and JC Norcross. 1992. In search of how people change: applications to addictive behaviors. *Am J Psychol.* 47:1102-1114.

Rimer, BK, CT Orleans, MK Keintz et al. 1990. The older smoker: status, challenges, and opportunities for intervention. *Chest.* 97(3)547-553.

Sachs, DPL. 1986. Cigarette smoking: health effects and cessation strategies. *Clinics in Ger Med.* 2:337-362.

Speizer, FE and IB Tager. 1979. Epidemiology of chronic mucus hypersecretion and obstructive airways disease. *Epidemiol Rev.* 1:124-142.

Tillman, M and J Silcock. 1997. A comparison of smokers' and ex-smokers' health related quality of life. *J Publ Hlth Med.* 19(3):268-273.

US Dept of Health and Human Services. 1990. *The Health Benefits of Smoking Cessation: a Report of the Surgeon General.* (DHHS publication No. [CDC] 90-8416) Bethesda: Office on Smoking and Health.

———. 1991. *Strategies to Control Tobacco Use in the United States: a Blueprint for Public Health Action in the 1990's.* 8-11. (NIH Publication No. 92-3316) Bethesda: National Cancer Institute.

US Dept of Health and Human Services, Centers for Disease Control and Prevention. 1998. Tobacco use among high school students—United States, 1997. *MMWR.* 47(12):229-233.

Vetter, NJ and D Ford. 1990. Smoking prevention among people aged 60 and older: a randomized clinical trial. *Aging.* 19:164-168.

Woodson, K, JA Tangrea, MJ Barrett et al. 1999. Serum apha-tocopherol and subsequent risk of lung cancer among male smokers. *J Nat Cancer Inst.* 91(20):1738-1743.

11

COPD and Osteoporosis

Diane M. Biskobing, MD

As chronic obstructive pulmonary disease (COPD) progresses and the patient becomes more debilitated, osteoporosis is a frequent finding (Iqbal 1999, Shane 1996). With progressive loss of bone mass the patient is at a high risk of suffering a vertebral or hip fracture. Fractures cause significant morbidity and even mortality in the already compromised patient. While fractures are more often seen in patients with advanced COPD, recognition of the problem and preventive measures should be instituted early in the disease process before fractures occur.

Frequency of Osteoporosis in COPD Patients

Low Bone Mineral Density

Osteoporosis is characterized by low bone mass accompanied by microarchitectural changes in bone, increasing susceptibility to fracture. The World Health Organization definition for osteoporosis is based on measurement of bone mineral density (BMD). Osteopenia is defined as a BMD between 1 and 2.5 standard deviations below the young adult mean while osteoporosis is defined as a BMD more than 2.5 standard deviations below the young adult mean (Eastell 1998).

As many as 35% to 72% of patients with COPD have been reported to be osteopenic and 36% to 49% have osteoporosis (Iqbal 1999, Shane 1996). As the severity of COPD progresses, the proportion of patients with osteoporosis increases (Iqbal 1999, McEvoy 1998). Praet et al (1992) studied BMD in men with chronic bronchitis. Vertebral BMD was lower than age-matched controls in all patients studied, irrespective of glucocorticoid exposure. In a similar study by del Pino-Montes et al (1999) both hip and spine BMD were significantly lower in a group of men with COPD without prior exposure to glucocorticoids compared with age-matched controls. In a group of male subjects at a VA Medical Center, subjects with chronic lung disease were five times more likely to have osteoporosis than control patients with hypertension (Iqbal 1999). Increased risk was seen in subjects with no previous exposure to oral or inhaled corticosteroids. The subjects with more severe compromise in lung function who used inhaled or oral glucocorticoids had a nine-fold increased risk of osteoporosis. The risk did not change with inhaled versus oral glucocorticoids (Iqbal 1999).

Decreased BMD has been reported with both inhaled and oral corticosteroids. The loss in BMD is generally less with inhaled glucocorticoids compared with oral steroids. Ebeling et al (1998) and Marystone et al (1995) both described BMD in users of inhaled steroids intermediate between users of oral steroids and those never exposed to glucocorticoids. However, both Toogood et al (1995) and Wisniewski et al (1997) reported a dose-dependent decrease in BMD with inhaled glucocorticoids. For each 1 mg/d of inhaled steroid, BMD fell by about 5% relative to the age-matched normal reference range (Toogood 1995). The authors also reported improved BMD with a higher lifetime dose of inhaled steroids and concluded that the higher BMD resulted from less exposure to oral glucocorticoids. In summary, inhaled glucocorticoids produce less bone loss than oral but, over an extended time period, can still produce significant bone loss.

Biochemical Changes in Bone Metabolism

Changes in bone metabolism can be measured with biochemical markers, which include the bone formation markers *osteocalcin* and *bone specific alkaline phosphatase*. The biochemical marker osteocalcin was lower than a control in men with chronic bronchitis, with or without a history of glucocorticoid use (Praet 1992), suggesting decreased bone formation in the chronically ill patients. In the setting of glucocorticoid use, decreased osteocalcin and bone specific alkaline phosphatase, implying impaired bone formation, is well documented (Ebeling 1998, Hodsman 1991, Lukert and Raisz 1990). The decrease in bone formation markers is seen with either inhaled or oral glucocorticoids (Ebeling 1998, Hodsman 1991).

Vitamin D deficiency also appears to play a role in the declining BMD associated with COPD. Riancho et al (1987) reported significantly decreased 25-hydroxyvitamin D levels in a group of men with COPD not taking chronic glucocorticoids compared with control subjects of similar age. The authors documented a correlation between sun exposure and the 25-hydroxyvitamin D level. In a group of patients with severe lung disease awaiting lung transplantation, 35% of the COPD patients had markedly low 25-hydroxyvitamin D levels ($\leq$ 10 ng/ml) (Shane 1996). Thus, vitamin D deficiency may contribute to the decreased BMD associated with COPD due to less sun exposure as a result of decreased functional status.

Fractures

Low bone mass per se is asymptomatic and causes no morbidity. However, the consequences of osteoporosis—fractures—can cause significant debility. Thoracic vertebral fractures may further compromise lung function

(Leech 1990, Lisboa 1985) and hip fractures decrease mobility and are associated with significant mortality (Myers 1991).

Vertebral fractures are often asymptomatic and may seem of little significance. However, the fractures that are symptomatic can cause significant morbidity because of pain. This pain can be distressing to a patient who is already struggling to breathe. In addition, with progressive kyphosis due to thoracic vertebral fractures, further loss of lung volume may have devastating consequences for the patient with COPD. In a study of a group of nine patients with severe kyphoscoliosis who were nonsmokers, forced vital capacity (FVC) was 29% predicted and total lung capacity, 44% predicted (Lisboa 1985). In addition, respiratory muscle function was significantly impaired. In a study of women with osteoporosis, each thoracic vertebral fracture decreased FVC by approximately 9% (Leech 1990). While this may have a minimal effect on someone with normal lung function, the effect on someone with COPD may be significant.

The prevalence of vertebral fractures in patients with COPD has been reported to be increased compared with the normal population. In a study of patients awaiting lung transplantation the prevalence rate was 29% (Shane 1996). Another study of patients with COPD revealed a prevalence of vertebral fractures of 49% in patients who had never taken any glucocorticoids to as high as 63% in those on systemic glucocorticoids (McEvoy 1998). Thoracic vertebral fractures were more common than lumbar fractures in all patients. Multiple fractures were more common in the systemic steroid users. However, another group reported no increase in vertebral fractures in patients with COPD without a history of chronic glucocorticoid use (Riancho 1987).

Hip fractures are the most serious outcome of osteoporosis. The risk for hip fracture is increased with decreased BMD and also increases with the presence of one or more chronic conditions (Mussolino 1998). Hip fractures have significant morbidity, often resulting in decreased mobility and independence for the patient (Cooper and Melton 1995). In the severely dyspneic COPD patient, further loss of mobility after a hip fracture may lead to increased dependence on the caretaker. Many patients require nursing home care after hip fracture due to the loss of independence (Cooper and Melton 1995). In addition there is an increased mortality rate after hip fracture. Overall in-hospital mortality after a hip fracture for patients over 65 years of age was 4.9% (Myers 1991), and mortality is as much as 2 times greater in males than females. As the number of other medical diagnoses increases, mortality increases as well (Myers 1991).

Pathophysiology of Osteoporosis in COPD Patients

There are numerous risk factors that contribute to the pathophysiology of osteoporosis seen in COPD patients, which include glucocorticoid treatment, smoking and alcohol abuse, low body mass index (BMI), and immobility as the disease progresses. Of these, the use of glucocorticoids is the most significant. However, since osteoporosis has been reported in COPD patients without any history of corticosteroid use, the other risk factors as well must play a significant role in the progression of the disease.

Glucocorticoids

Glucocorticoid-induced osteoporosis is well-documented in the literature. Patients on high doses of glucocorticoids exhibit a rapid loss of BMD within the first 6 months. The mechanism is two-fold: decreased bone formation and increased bone resorption. Bone formation is decreased through inhibition of osteoblast function (Canalis 1996). This has been demonstrated on histomorphometic analysis of bone biopsies (Dempster 1989) and with decreased levels of osteocalcin, a biochemical marker of bone formation (Ebeling 1998, Hodsman 1991, Lukert and Raisz 1990). The accelerated bone resorption seen with the use of glucocorticoids appears to be due to secondary hyperparathyroidism. Glucocorticoids decrease intestinal calcium absorption and increase urinary calcium excretion, causing a rise in PTH levels that stimulates bone resorption. The elevation in PTH activates osteoclasts and accelerates bone resorption (Adachi 1997, Lukert and Raisz 1990). Until recently, the effects of corticosteroids on bone metabolism were thought to occur only with oral steroids. However, suppression of osteocalcin levels has been documented both with oral and inhaled glucocorticoids (Ebeling 1998, Hodsman 1991). Decreased bone density as well has been documented in patients on oral or inhaled glucocorticoids (Ebeling 1998, Marystone 1995).

Glucocorticoids can also cause hypogonadism in both men and women (Adachi 1997, Lukert and Raisz 1990). Corticosteroid use decreases gonadotropin secretion from the pituitary. In addition, estrogen or testosterone production is decreased in response to leutenizing hormone. These combined effects result in hypogonadism. If left untreated this will result in accelerated bone resorption as well. All men and premenopausal women should be monitored for development of hypogonadism and put on replacement therapy if indicated. In postmenopausal women, hormone replacement therapy should be instituted.

Smoking and Alcohol Use

Smoking has been shown to be an independent risk factor for osteoporosis in both men and women (Daniell 1976, Seeman 1983, Sparrow 1982). Slemenda et al (1989) showed lower BMD in heavy smokers compared with nonsmokers. Several groups (Krall and Dawson-Hughes 1991, Slemenda 1992, Sparrow 1982) have demonstrated significantly greater rate of bone loss in smokers compared with nonsmokers, and both vertebral fractures and hip fractures are increased in smokers (Cooper 1988, Daniell 1976,

Seeman 1983). Seeman et al (1983) reported a 2.3-fold increased risk of vertebral fracture among smokers. The authors, however, found this relationship only in long-term smokers. Cooper et al (1988) reported a 1.7-fold increased risk for hip fracture among smokers. The pathophysiologic mechanism for the lower bone mass and increased fracture risk in smokers is unclear. Some studies have suggested that estrogen levels are lower in smokers compared to nonsmokers (Seeman 1996). One study has shown decreased calcium absorption in the gastrointestinal tract in smokers compared with nonsmokers (Krall and Dawson-Hughes 1991).

Excessive alcohol use has also been associated with increased rates of osteoporosis and fracture. The rate of bone loss has been shown to be associated with the amount of alcohol use, ie, a greater rate of bone loss is seen in those who consume higher amounts of alcohol (Slemenda 1992). Both increased vertebral and hip fracture risks are associated with excessive alcohol use. The direct effects of alcohol on osteoblast function lead to decreased bone formation (Seeman 1996). In addition, poor nutrition, hypogonadism, vitamin D deficiency, and liver disease may also contribute to lower BMD in these patients. The markedly increased fracture rate in men with a history of alcohol abuse is most likely related to increased falls.

The combined use of tobacco and alcohol markedly increases the risk of osteoporosis. Slemenda et al (1992) demonstrated the highest rate of bone loss in those with high alcohol and tobacco use, and the risk for vertebral fracture is markedly increased as well in those who both smoke and drink alcohol. In nonobese smokers and drinkers aged 60-69 years the relative risk for vertebral fracture was 3; in those aged 70 year and older, the relative risk increased to 20.2 (Seeman 1983).

Body Mass Index

Bone mass is directly correlated with BMI. Both men and women with high BMI have higher BMD. This is thought to be due partially to the effect of greater weight-bearing load on the bones (Cauley 1996). In addition, estrogen levels tend to be higher in obese people due to increased aromitization of testosterone to estrogen in the adipose tissue (Cauley 1996). The resulting higher estradiol levels may help explain the higher BMD in the obese since estradiol levels in both men and women correlate with BMD (Greendale 1997, Khosla 1998). Many patients with end-stage COPD lose weight as the disease progresses. Iqbal et al (1999) reported the lowest BMD was seen in a group of patients with BMI below the normal median.

Immobility

Normal weight-bearing activity has been shown to be required for maintenance of bone mass. Complete immobilization, such as paralysis or in experimental settings, has been shown to accelerate bone turnover, resulting in decreased BMD (Gambert 1995, Kiratli 1996). Most patients with COPD are not completely immobilized; however, advanced COPD is often associated with decreased functional status and mobility. The decreased activity may increase the risk of falls and fracture since several case-control studies have demonstrated an inverse correlation between hip fracture risk and amount of daily activities. Cooper et al (1988) evaluated daily activity and grip strength in a case-control study of patients with hip fractures and found that a decrease in activities such as standing, walking, stair climbing, and housework was associated with significantly increased risk for hip fracture. Decreased grip strength was shown to be an independent risk factor for hip fracture.

Prevention and Treatment

Prevention of osteoporosis in patients with COPD is dependent on an awareness of the magnitude of the problem. Since patients are generally asymptomatic until they suffer a fracture, there is little impetus for screening and/or preventive therapy. However, early recognition and institution of preventive therapy is essential to avoid complications such as fractures. Because of the high incidence of osteopenia and osteoporosis in the COPD population and documented low levels of 25-hydroxyvitamin D, all COPD patients should be put on calcium and vitamin D supplements.

It has been suggested that all patients with COPD should be screened for measurement of BMD (Iqbal 1999). While the screening of all patients is controversial, the evidence supports the recommendation. The prevalence of osteoporosis in those with COPD, irrespective of treatment, is similar to that seen in postmenopausal women. The prevalence in COPD patients reported ranged between 36% and 49%, whereas the prevalence of osteoporosis in postmenopausal women has been reported to be approximately 35% (Melton 1998). These numbers would support screening all patients so as to identify those with osteoporosis and at a high risk of fracture.

Nonpharmacologic therapies can be beneficial in the prevention and treatment of osteoporosis in all patients with COPD. Evidence of decreased muscle strength and balance, such as the inability to rise from a chair, slow gait speed, and decreased grip strength, have been shown to be associated with an increased risk of hip fracture (Cooper 1988, Cummings 1995). A physical therapy program designed to increase exercise endurance, muscle strength, and balance will not only improve the functional status and quality of life but will also decrease the risk of falling and subsequent fractures (McClung and Spencer 1996).

Since steroid-induced bone loss occurs very early in the course of treatment, COPD patients who are being started on inhaled or oral glucocorticoids should be considered for preventive therapy. As discussed previously, all patients should be taking calcium and vitamin D supplements. Calcium and vitamin D alone, however, are generally insufficient to prevent the bone loss associated with high dose glucocorticoid treatment (Sambrook 1993). There is now substantial evidence that initiation of a bisphosphonate when glucocorticoids are begun will prevent significant loss of BMD. In a randomized study of 141 patients beginning long-term glucocorticoid treatment for rheumatologic diseases, intermittent etidronate, when started within 3 months, prevented bone loss, as compared with 500 mg of calcium alone (Adachi 1996). In a similar study of alendronate versus 800 to 1000 mg of calcium and 250 to 500 IU of vitamin D, alendronate significantly increased BMD compared with the calcium and vitamin D group (Saag 1998). While these studies were mainly in patients with rheumatologic diseases, they provide strong evidence that bisphosphonates can prevent steroid-induced bone loss. There is also evidence that bisphosphonates can improve BMD in patients who already have bone loss due to glucocorticoids. In a smaller treatment study of 49 patients on glucocorticoids for 6 months or more, patients were randomized to intermittent etidronate plus calcium versus placebo plus calcium. BMD in the placebo-treated patients stayed stable whereas BMD in the etidronate group rose 4%. Forty-three percent of the patients in the study were asthmatics (Pitt 1998). There are only a few small studies specifically addressing osteoporosis treatment in patients with lung disease. One study by Gallacher et al (1992) of asthmatic patients treated with steroids demonstrated increased lumbar BMD in response to cyclic pamidronate infusions. Based on the results, patients on long term (> 3 months) oral glucocorticoids should be treated with a bisphosphonate. The more difficult issue is whether patients on inhaled glucocorticoids should be placed on any preventive therapy. There are no studies that specifically address this issue. Since the bone loss from inhaled glucocorticoids is generally less than that seen with oral steroids, more conservative management may be adequate as long as patients are followed closely with measurement of BMD.

Summary

Osteoporosis and subsequent fractures are common problems in patients with COPD. Fractures can produce significant comorbidity in such patients. While the use of glucocorticoids increases the frequency of osteoporosis, the problem is also seen in patients not treated with glucocorticoids. Awareness of the problem and strategies to prevent development of osteoporosis during the course of COPD therapy is essential to decrease the incidence of fractures in these patients.

References

Adachi, JD. 1997. Corticosteroid-induced osteoporosis. *Am J Med Sci.* 313(1):41-49.

Adachi, JD, WG Bensen, F Bianchi et al. 1996. Vitamin D and calcium in the prevention of corticosteroid induced osteoporosis: a 3-year followup. *J Rheumatology*. 23:995-1000.

Canalis, E. 1996. Mechanisms of glucocorticoid action in bone: implications to glucocorticoid-induced osteoporosis. *J Clin Endocrin & Metabol*. 81(10):3441-3447.

Cauley, JA, LM Salamone, and FL Lucas. 1996. Postmenopausal endogenous and exogenous hormones, degree of obesity, thiazide diuretics, and risk of osteoporosis. In *Osteoporosis*, eds. R Marcus, D Feldman, and J Kelsey, 551-576. Academic Press.

Cooper, C, DJ Barker, and C Wickham. 1988. Physical activity, muscle strength, and calcium intake in fracture of the proximal femur in Britain. *Brit Med J*. 297:1443-1446.

Cooper, C and LJ Melton. 1995. Magnitude and impact of osteoporosis and fractures. In *Osteoporosis*, eds. R Marcus, D Feldman, and J Kelsey, 419-434. Academic Press.

Cummings, SR, MC Nevitt, WS Browner et al. 1995. Risk factors for hip fracture in white women. *New Eng J Med*. 332:767-773.

Daniell, HW. 1976. Osteoporosis of the slender smoker. *Arch Int Med*. 136:298-304.

del Pino-Montes, J, JL Fernandez, F Gomez et al. 1999. *Bone mineral density is related to emphysema and lung function in chronic obstructive pulmonary disease*. Paper presented at the annual meeting of the American Society for Bone and Mineral Research, St. Louis, MO (Sep 30-Oct 4).

Dempster, DW. 1989. Bone histomorphometry in glucocorticoid-induced osteoporosis. *J Bone & Mineral Research*. 4:137-141.

Eastell, R. 1998. Treatment of postmenopausal osteoporosis. *New Eng J Med*. 338(11):736-746.

Ebeling, PR, B Erbas, J Hopper et al. 1998. Bone mineral density and bone turnover in asthmatics treated with long-term inhaled or oral glucocorticoids. *J Bone & Mineral Research*. 12:1283-1289.

———. 1998. Bone mineral density and bone turnover in asthmatics treated with long-term inhaled or oral glucocorticoids. *J Bone & Mineral Research*. 13:1283-1289.

Gallacher, SJ, JA Fenner, K Anderson et al. 1992. Intravenous pamidronate in the treatment of osteoporosis associated with corticosteroid dependent lung disease: an open pilot study. *Thorax*. 47:932-936.

Gambert, SR, BM Schultz, and RC Hamdy. 1995. Osteoporosis: clinical features, prevention, and treatment. *Endocrin & Metabol Clinics of North Amer*. 24:317-371.

Greendale, GA, S Edelstein, and CE Barrett. 1997. Endogenous sex steroids and bone mineral density in older women and men: the Rancho Bernardo Study. *J Bone & Mineral Research*. 12(11):1833-1843.

Hodsman, AB, JH Toogood, B Jennings et al. 1991. Differential effects of inhaled budesonide and oral prednisolone on serum osteocalcin. *J Clin Endocrin & Metabol*. 72:530-540.

Iqbal, F, J Michaelson, L Thaler et al. 1999. Declining bone mass in men with chronic pulmonary disease: contribution of glucocorticoid treatment, body mass index, and gonadal function. *Chest*. 116(6): 1616-1624.

Khosla, S, LJ Melton, E Atkinson et al. 1998. Relationship of serum sex steroid levels and bone turnover markers with bone mineral density in men and women: a key role for bioavailable estrogen. *J Clin Endocrin & Metabol.* 83(7):2266-2274.

Kiratli, BJ. 1996. Immobilization osteopenia. In *Osteoporosis*, eds. R Marcus, D Feldman, and J Kelsey, 833-853. Academic Press.

Krall, EA and B Dawson-Hughes. 1991. Smoking and bone loss among postmenopausal women. *J Bone & Mineral Research.* 6(4):331-337.

Leech, JA, C Dulberg, S Kellie et al. 1990. Relationship of lung function to severity of osteoporosis in women. *Am Review Respir Dis.* 141:68-71.

Lisboa, C, R Moreno, M Fava et al. 1985. Inspiratory muscle function in patients with severe kyphoscoliosis. *Am Review Respir Dis.* 132:48-52.

Lukert, BP and LG Raisz. 1990. Glucocorticoid-induced osteoporosis: pathogenesis and management. *Annals Int Med.* 112:352-364.

Marystone, JF, EL Barrett-Connor, and DJ Morton. 1995. Inhaled and oral coricosteroids: their effects on bone mineral density in older adults. *Am J Pub Hlth.* 85:1693-1695.

McClung, MR and K Spencer. 1996. Nonpharmacologic therapy for osteoporosis. In *Osteoporosis: Diagnostic and Therapeutic Principles*, ed. CJ Rosen, 189-199. Humana Press.

McEvoy, C, K Ensrud, E Bender et al. 1998. Association between coricosteroid use and vertebral fractures in older men with chronic obstructive pulmonary disease. *Am J Respir & Crit Care Med.* 157:704-709.

Melton LJ, EJ Atkinson, MK O'Connor et al. 1998. Bone density and fracture risk in men. *J Bone & Mineral Research.* 13(12):1915-1923.

Mussolino, ME, AC Looker, JH Madans et al. 1998. Risk factors for hip fracture in white men: the NHANES I epidemiologic follow-up study. *J Bone & Mineral Research.* 13(6):918-924.

Myers, AH, EG Robinson, ML Van Natta et al. 1991. Hip fractures among the elderly: factors associated with in-hospital mortality. *Am J Epidemiology.* 134:1128-1137.

Pitt, P, F Li, P Todd et al. 1998. A double blind placebo controlled study to determine the effects of intermittent cyclical etidronate on bone mineral density in patients on long term oral corticosteroid treatment. *Thorax.* 53:351-356.

Praet, JP, A Peretz, S Rozenberg et al. 1992. Risk of osteoporosis in men with chronic bronchitis. *Osteoporosis Intl.* 2:257-261.

Riancho, JA, JG Macias, C Del Arco et al. 1987. Vertebral compression fractures and mineral metabolism in chronic obstructive lung disease. *Thorax.* 42:962-966.

Saag, KG, R Emkey, TJ Schnitzer et al. 1998. Alendronate for the prevention and treatment of glucocorticoid-induced osteoporosis. *New Eng J Med.* 339:292-299.

Sambrook, P, J Birmingham, P Kelly et al. 1993. Prevention of corticosteroid osteoporosis: a comparison of calcium, calcitriol, and calcitonin. *New Eng J Med.* 328(24):1747-1752.

Seeman, E. 1996. The effects of tobacco and alcohol use on bone. In *Osteoporosis*, eds. R Marcus, D Feldman, and J Kelsey, 577-597. Academic Press.

Seeman, E, LJ Melton, WM O'Fallon, and BL Riggs. 1983. Risk factors for spinal osteoporosis in men. *Am J Med.* 75:977-983.

Shane, E, SJ Silverberg, D Donovan et al. 1996. Osteoporosis in lung transplantation candidates with end-stage pulmonary disease. *Am J Med*. 101:262-269.

Slemenda, CW, JC Christian, T Reed et al. 1992. Long-term bone loss in men: effects of genetic and environmental factors. *Annals Int Med*. 117:286-291.

Slemenda, CW, SL Hui, C Longcope, and CC Johnston. 1989. Cigarette smoking, obesity, and bone mass. *J Bone & Mineral Research*. 4(5):737-741.

Sparrow, D, NI Beausoleil, AJ Garvey et al. 1982. The influence of cigarette smoking and age on bone loss in men. *Arch Environ Hlth*. 37:246-249.

Toogood, JH, JC Baskerville, AE Markov et al. 1995. Bone mineral density and the risk of fracture in patients receiving long-term inhaled steroid therapy for asthma. *J Allergy & Clin Immun*. 96(157):166.

Wisniewski, AF, SA Lewis, DJ Green et al. 1997. Cross sectional investigation of the effects of inhaled corticosteroids on bone density and bone metabolism in patients with asthma. *Thorax*. 52:853-860.

12

Self-Help Groups for Life-Threatening Illnesses: Support for Behavior Change

Hannah L. Hedrick, PhD, and Daryl Holtz Isenberg, PhD

> *Company is better than will power*
> *when you are trying to change behavior.*
> —Amrit Desai

While people may join a self-help group for information about and support for their common situation or condition, they frequently receive an unanticipated benefit: encouragement and support in improving their general health and quality of life throughout their recovery or illness. The techniques used to help members cope with their common condition—sharing stories, offering constructive advice, and mentoring—are also useful in assisting members in replacing unhealthy habits.

Almost all groups offer some techniques for helping members with changes related to the specific condition that drew them to the group. Recovery (12 step) groups are known for their success in using a sponsor system to help members stop drinking, using drugs, overeating, etc. Some groups go beyond help in stopping abusive behavior to offering support in achieving a healthier lifestyle. For example, Parents Anonymous focuses not only on stopping abuse but also on specific techniques to deal with stress. Groups for stroke and diabetes are exemplary in their disease prevention efforts, frequently related to diet and physical activity.

The self-care benefits derived from group participation were acknowledged in the September 1989 issue of *Population Reports*. Groups for AIDS/HIV were credited with providing the "knowledge, emotions, and skills [that] reinforce healthful changes," permitting "people to change their behavior and to maintain new behavior."

The "Helper-Therapy" Principle

How can participating in a self-help group bring about changes that nagging family and friends could not create? Part of the success comes from the peer aspect—the sponsor or buddy knows exactly how difficult it is to "just say no," or to get out of bed to go for a walk, or even to leave the house or bedroom. Having someone who has "been there" hold your hand (literally) or listen to you cry at 2:00 am also helps. Groups frequently provide a forum for sharing stories of struggle and success, convincing other members that they, too, can improve the quality of their life by making better choices and acting on them. Seeing others succeed in giving up that pint of ice cream at bedtime, in dancing around the room or doing deep breathing when they feel like having a cigarette, or in shopping and cooking together to avoid dietary no-no's is evidence that it can be done. The intimacy developed during these shared activities or even just talking about them also can reduce stress that exacerbates symptoms in many life-threatening illnesses.

The encouragement and company of one who has "been there" is no doubt highly motivational. But another attribute of self-help groups also contributes to long-term behavior change. Having opportunities to use your experience to help others is one of the major benefits provided by groups. And one way to help is to keep someone company in a healthy activity. Members are less likely to sit in front of the TV and reach for another beer or pretzel when they have promised a self-help group friend to do t'ai chi chih or yoga with them or take them to a massage therapist.

Numerous studies have shown how the benefits of altruism accrue to the giver as well as the receiver. The personal inconvenience members sometimes endure, whether helping with the condition that draws members together or helping members assume more control over their lives, is a prime example of altruism.

Group Mechanisms for Promoting Health

In addition to offering members a forum for sharing success stories and strategies, groups for life-threatening illnesses may have structured mechanisms for encouraging members to assume responsibility for retaining and maintaining a healthy lifestyle. Among the most common are presentations, demonstrations, and ongoing programs on movement techniques, food choices, stress reduction, and other self-care techniques that can improve general health.

The widely published works of researchers Dean Ornish and Meyer Friedman indicate that the mind can modify behavior, altering the course of heart disease. Ornish's study demonstrated the positive effect of support group training. Lawrence LeShan achieved similarly impressive improvements from helping cancer patients access repressed negative emotions. Neuroscientist Candace Pert has helped us understand the roles of neuropeptides and how emotions and health are connected at the molecular level: "Emotions are a key element in self-care because they allow us to enter into the body-mind conversation and direct them through the psychosomatic network" (1997, p. 283). Elmer Green, a scientist who quantifies the practical value of meditative states, provides a measurable technology, biofeedback, for accessing an inner intelligence: "We have been inhibited, repressed, and hypnotized by our cultural conditioning and education to see ourselves as powerless to control or change events in our bodies and lives.

We have not been informed that our bodies tend to do what they are told to do if we know how to tell them. Only when we do not accept this limiting image of ourselves can we break the thralldom and begin to operate as free beings, capable of influencing to a significant extent the course of our lives" (from a conversation cited in Schwartz 1995, pp. 117-118).

These body/mind interventions are believed by the above authors to be as potent as diet, drug, or exercise. Self-help groups, with their spontaneous and adaptive responses to human needs, frequently use body/mind interventions to accomplish their goal of empowering people to take charge of their lives. In summary, self-help groups provide a number of activities that support these interventions:

- Members informally link each other to sources of support for healthy behaviors, including complementary health care services.
- Groups incorporate health-inducing activities, such as t'ai chi chih, art therapy, massage, journaling, meditation, guided imagery, nutrition, and pet therapy, as well as support for spiritual development.
- Groups conduct ongoing peer-led programs or sponsor professional presenters.
- Professionals and self-help group members can co-facilitate body/mind interventions. The founder of AA is well known; other professionals who emphasize the importance of peer support in helping people with life-threatening illnesses change their behavior include Jerry Jampolsky, MD (Center for Attitudinal Healing); Bernie Siegel, MD (the Exceptional Cancer Patient program); Dean Ornish, MD (includes peer support in his program to reverse heart disease); Simon Stephens, MDiv (bereavement program encourages parent-to-parent communication); and Con Keogh, MDiv (developed Grow, International to bring together people affected by chronic mental illness).

Self-help groups are likely to be on their own when figuring out how to support self-care and health promotion activities. Although the International Information Centre on Self-Help and Health pointed out a decade ago that the health care system should provide support for groups ready to undertake these roles, systematic support has not yet been provided.

Complementary Health Care Systems and Practices

Some health care professionals and others are concerned that the self-care and health promotion activities presented in self-help group settings may not be adequately tested for safety and efficacy. They are especially concerned about practices labeled as "alternative" or "complementary," referring to interventions for improving, maintaining, and promoting health and well-being, preventing disease, or treating illnesses that are not usually part of a standard North American biomedical regimen of health care or disease prevention. In fact, "self-help groups" themselves have been included in lists of such practices.

Groups for life-threatening illnesses, especially those in the advanced stages, are well known for their willingness to consider nonbiomedical practices to assist in symptom control. As Wayne Jonas, MD, comments in "Alternative Medicine: Learning from the Past, Advancing to the Future" (*Journal of the American Medical Association*, November 1998), "Alternative medicine is here to stay. It is no longer an option to ignore it or treat it as something outside the normal processes of science and medicine."

But many professionals are still apprehensive about the ways in which self-help groups present complementary health practices. The perception persists in some quarters that the information disseminated by lay-led organizations is anti-medical and even injurious, although research results on the safety and efficacy of some complementary health care practices and of approaches used by self-help groups have partially alleviated those fears and suspicions. Research results published in the *Journal of the American Medical Association* (*JAMA*) in August 1999 indicate that less then 2% of users of complementary health care modalities avoid allopathic treatments. Professional concerns are also alleviated by the knowledge that self-help groups now have electronic access to information about the efficacy and safety of conventional as well as complementary practices.

Moreover, self-help groups in general have mechanisms to avoid undue influence on members to use "unproven" and potentially "unsafe" practices. In addition to offering a platform for proponents of the treatment, groups usually invite members to share their opinions and experiences. The opinions of members with considerable positive experience in and knowledge about self-care and complementary practices are balanced by the healthy skepticism of other members. This "wisdom of the group" provides a unique filter of personal testimony that assists members in deciding for themselves whether or not to try a general or specific remedy. Even groups that regularly present information about a wide variety of self-care and complementary modalities rarely give blanket approval to any modalities about which efficacy and safety are issues. In any event, most complementary health care practices are noninvasive and therefore relatively safe.

Increasing evidence of the safety and efficacy of many complementary health care practices has been provided through research supported by the National Center for Complementary and Alternative Medicine, established by the National Institutes of Health. National consensus conferences, such as the 1997 conference announcing the effectiveness of acupuncture for some conditions, have reversed skepticism about some common practices. Numerous policies, reports, and publications had presented irrefutable evidence that (1) respectful communication about patient preferences and practices is crucial for adherence to biomedical treatment and (2) health care belief systems are critical to the patient's healing process. At the same time, schools of medicine, nursing, and other health professions have added or are adding curriculum in areas such as mind/body interventions, nonbiomedical systems, diet and nutrition, bioelectromagnetic applications, manual healing techniques, and herbal medicines and remedies.

Self-help group members confronted by end-stage illnesses may also choose to use complementary practices simply because they are part of their family or national background or because they believe such practices are less harmful than biomedicine. The emphasis of managed care organizations on low-risk interventions, self-care, and prevention also appears to be boosting interest in and increasing access to nonbiomedical treatments. An increasing number of clinics, group practices, and other settings are offering multiple modalities through an "integrative medicine" unit. Varied options for reimbursement are available through insurance companies and managed care plans. This trend is likely to continue as mainstream publications, such as the November 1998 issues of *JAMA* and the *AMA Archives* journals, report the results of clinical studies demonstrating the efficacy and cost-effectiveness of specific techniques.

Of particular relevance to self-help groups and advanced-stage illnesses is the increasing attention given to spiritual beliefs and practices in connection with "comfort care" and decision making at the end of life. Studies also suggest an association between spiritual practices and improved outcomes in nonterminal situations. Herbert Benson, MD, has declared that spiritual practices clearly complement traditional medicine and that "we should make every effort to incorporate our patient's spirituality to promote healing" (Mark Moran, *AMNews*, April 12, 1999). Since 1997, the National Institute for Healthcare Research and the John Templeton Foundation have awarded grants to 19 medical schools to develop curricula in spirituality and medicine. More than 50 US medical schools now offer elective courses in spirituality. A number of annual symposia have been established by the Annenberg Center for Health Sciences, National Institute for Healthcare Research, and Association of American Medical Colleges, and annual meetings of the American Public Health Association include many presentations related to spirituality and health care.

Selected Complementary Health Care Systems and Practices

The following categories and selected complementary health care systems and practices are presented only to indicate the variety of modalities that may be available to members of self-help groups for persons with life-threatening illnesses. The list is not to be used to indicate any type of recognition or endorsement of any of the categories or selected practices by any self-help group. Some categories have similar entries. For example, spirituality is included as a mind/body intervention (prayer and mental healing) and as a nonbiomedical system (anthroposophic medicine).

Mind/Body Interventions

Aromatherapy
Art therapy
Biofeedback
Dance/movement therapy
Hypnosis
Imagery
Meditation
Music therapy
Prayer and mental healing
Qigong
Self-help/support groups
T'ai chi chih/chuan
Writing therapy
Yoga

Systems (Nonbiomedical)

Acupuncture
Anthroposophic medicine
Ayurveda
Hispanic community health care
Homeopathy
Native American health care
Naturopathy
Traditional Oriental/Chinese
  medicine

Diet and Nutrition

Cultural diets
- Macrobiotic
- Mediterranean
- Traditional Native American
Diet modification regimens
- Amino acids
- Enzymes
- Minerals
- Supplemental therapies
- Vitamins (eg, antioxidants)

Bioelectromagnetic Applications

Electroacupuncture
Neuromagnetic stimulation
Transcranial electrostimulation

Manual or Energy Techniques

Biofield therapeutics
- Healing touch
- Polarity therapy
- Reiki
- SHEN physioemotional release therapy
- Therapeutic touch
Chiropractic/massage-related techniques
- Deep tissue massage
- Manual lymph drainage
- Neuromuscular massage
Postural reeducation
- Alexander technique
- Feldenkrais method
Pressure point therapies
Trager psychophysical integration

Herbal Medicines and Remedies

European botanical medicines
Latin American herbal remedies
Native American herbal agents
Oriental herbal agents
- Chinese
- Japanese-Kampo

Pharmacologic and Biologic Treatment Agents

Antineoplastons
Bee venom
Cartilage products

Ethylene diamine tetraacetic acid (EDTA) chelation therapy
Hoxsey method
Immunoaugmentive therapy
Ozone therapy

Resources

Becu, M, N Becu, G Manzur, and S Kochen. 1993. Self-help epilepsy groups: an evaluation of effect on depression and schizophrenia. *Epilesia.* 34(5):841-845.

Fennel, P. 1995. CFS sociocultural influences and trauma: clinical considerations. *J Chronic Fatigue Syndrome,* Volume 1, Number 3/4, 159-173.

Galanter, M. 1988. Zealous self-help groups as adjuncts to psychiatric treatment: a study of Recovery, Inc. *Am J Psychiatry.* 145(10):1248-1253.

Gartner, A and F Reissman. 1984. *Self-Help in the Human Services.* San Francisco, CA: Jossey-Bass.

Isenberg, DH. 1981. *Coping with Cancer, Belief Systems and Support in Cancer Self-Help Groups.* Doctoral Dissertation, Northwestern University.

Katz, A and E Bender. 1990. Toward definitions and classifications of self-help groups, in *Helping One Another: Self-Help Groups in a Changing World.* Oakland, CA: Third Party Publishing.

Katz, A, H Hedrick et al. 1992. *Self-Help: Concepts and Applications.* Philadelphia, PA: Charles Press.

Kurtz, LF. 1988. Mutual aid for affective disorders: the Manic-Depressive and Depressive Association. *Am J Orthopsychiatry.* 58(1):152-155.

Lieberman, MA and LD Borman. 1993. *Self-Help Groups for Coping with Crisis.* San Francisco, CA: Jossey-Bass.

Nash, KB and DD Kramer. 1993. Self-help for sickle cell disease in African American communities. *J Applied Behav Sci.* 29(2):202-215.

Pert, C. 1997. *Molecules of Emotion.* New York, NY: Simon & Schuster.

Raiff, NR. 1988. Some health related outcomes of self-help participation, in *The Self-Help Revolution,* eds. A Gartner and F Riessman. New York, NY: Human Sciences Press.

Schwartz, T. 1995. *What Really Matters, Searching for Wisdom in America.* New York, NY: Bantam Books.

Spiegel, D, JR Bloom, HC Kraemer, and E Bottheil. 1989. The effect of psychosocial treatment on survival of patients with metastatic breast cancer. *Lancet.* Oct 14: 888-891.

Surgeon General's Workshop on Self-Help and Public Health. 1987. US Dept of Health and Human Services, Public Health Services, Health Resources and Services Administration.

13

Taking Control of Our Health and Medical Destiny

Thomas D. Whitman

I was diagnosed with chronic obstructive pulmonary disease (COPD) almost 18 years ago. It would be expected, according to the norm, that the disease would have progressed to the point of total incapacitation by now. However, that is not the case. While I am unable to work and perform most of the activities I previously undertook, I lead a very active and useful life. There are a number of reasons for this, one of which is the many caring people I have met along my journey. I firmly believe, however, that without self-intervention, I would not be alive today. I also believe that even earlier intervention could have slowed the progression of the disease.

When I was originally diagnosed with COPD in 1981, the usual medicines (theophylline, albuterol, ipratropium bromide, and Azmacort) were prescribed and I was told to quit smoking. Yes, I was a smoker. Also, in the early 1960s, I worked in a shipbuilding facility, with extensive exposure to asbestos, and later I spent 15 years in an automobile factory where I was exposed to a variety of irritants, including welding dust, smoke, and asbestos. You might say I was a prime candidate for lung disease.

At no time following the diagnosis was I counseled about the severity of COPD, the consequences, the chain of events to follow, or what I could expect. I did quit smoking after a while, but not until I had had bronchitis many times: I would contract bronchitis or an upper respiratory infection approximately every 6 weeks.

My first pulmonologist examined me in 1993, when I was scheduled for a total hip replacement because of an arthritic condition. He told me that the emphysema I had was so severe that I would have to have an epidural rather than a general anesthetic in order to have the operation; general anesthesia would be too risky. He took a chest x-ray and performed an informal breathing test to determine the condition of my lungs. He remarked to me that my primary physician had me on a good therapy program and I should continue to follow through with her. I still received no comprehensive testing or counseling.

My condition kept getting worse; finally, it started to affect my performance at work. At this point, I was an account manager for an electronics company and the daily pressures and physical requirements of the job made it nearly impossible for me to perform my regular duties. (Fortunately, I had very understanding superiors.) I did not realize the effects that stress had on COPD and that stress could rapidly escalate the disease's progression, as it did in my case. Many times I felt I was losing control of my life. I was frustrated and extremely fearful of what was happening to me.

In January 1997, I went to Michigan because my mother had passed away from emphysema. Returning from the very cold weather there, I again contracted bronchitis. That, coupled with the stress of losing my mother and being unable to satisfactorily perform my duties at work, nearly caused a breakdown.

My primary physician scheduled me for a variety of procedures, including blood tests, a stress test, a sonogram, an x-ray, a visit with a cardiologist, and—lo and behold—a pulmonary function test (PFT)! This was the first that I had heard of the test. By this time, I could walk only a few steps without stopping to rest. Because of my condition, it took the respiratory therapist nearly 3½ hours to conduct the PFT, which usually takes only 1 hour to perform. During the test, the therapist talked to me about pulmonary rehabilitation and her belief that it could improve the quality of my life. She also informed me of a facility nearby where I could get the therapy.

When the test results were examined they revealed, among many other things, an FEV_1 of 14% of predicted. Blood gases tests coupled with 24-hour oximeter testing determined that I required supplementary oxygen 24 hours a day, with a requirement of 2 l pm at rest and 4 l pm while ambulatory. My self-esteem was at its lowest point. The primary physician told me that unless I immediately changed my lifestyle, including removing the stress factors of the work environment and maintaining proper diet, adequate rest, and exercise, I would not live more than 1 or 2 years. It was apparent that no one was going to lead me by the hand through this, so I decided to take control of my health and medical destiny.

Taking Control

I requested and received permission from the primary physician to attend a rehabilitation program. I participated in a 10-week outpatient pulmonary rehabilitation program, whose regimen consisted of oxygen administration, nebulized bronchodilators, incentive spirometry, inspiratory muscle training, breathing training, physical conditioning, and endurance training. I also participated in education sessions that focused on the disease process, lifestyle modification, and treatments. I attended weekly behavioral medicine support sessions to enhance the skills necessary for me to cope with COPD. After a few sessions, I became determined to learn as much about COPD as I possibly could so that I would know what decisions to make in the future. The benefits derived from the rehabilitation program literally saved my life.

In the beginning of rehabilitation, I could barely perform the exercises; now, after 2½ years, I exercise *every* day. I have changed my diet and my health has improved to the point that my body is better conditioned than it has been in years. In general, my life has taken a dramatic turn. I understand that this is a lifelong commitment that I must make to myself. While I am unable to engage in many of the activities I used to, or deal with stress as before, I channel my energies into other areas, such as helping to educate others, increasing public awareness of COPD, and speaking out in an attempt to have more research monies allocated to COPD.

I also made an appointment with a new pulmonologist. His first reaction to my condition was: "Do you have children and do they understand how bad your condition is?" He was a very good physician, but appeared to want to treat the immediate problem only and send me on my way. He moved away shortly thereafter and assigned me to an associate in his practice.

In July 1998, I was hospitalized with a severe case of pneumonia and a collapsed lung. The pulmonologist to whom I was now assigned treated me and performed a bronchoscopy, and I pulled through after a lengthy recuperation period. Upon my return to some degree of stability, he released me, saying, "You're doing fine and I won't need to see you again until you have a problem." This was not the kind of comment I wanted to hear! While he is an excellent physician in my opinion and is still my pulmonologist, I would have liked to hear him say that he wanted to see me in 3 or 6 months to check on my condition and progress.

What if new medicines or treatments become available for COPD? Will either of the physicians call to inform me about them? The only way I will learn about them is if I find out about them myself. At no point has anyone discussed the possibility of lung volume reduction surgery or a lung transplant. However, following my own extensive reading, Internet research, and statistical evaluation, I have determined that because of the positive reaction I have had to my present therapy, these are options I would not consider at this time. No one is looking out for my welfare but *me*. I understand that caseloads are heavy and I appreciate the demands on a physician's time, but nevertheless there are some serious deficiencies here. *I* must keep *myself* informed and *I* remind the physicians about periodic blood work, new medicines, etc.

I feel that the medical community has let me down. Why did not someone suggest rehabilitation at a much earlier stage? Why am I not kept informed of new treatments? I realize that these things require time, but too many COPD patients are given standard treatments, made as comfortable as possible, and then ignored. At this point, many patients just give up and wait to succumb to the devastation of the disease.

I joined an on-line support group called E.F.F.O.R.T.S. (Emphysema Foundation for Our Right to Survive). The Web site has a large amount of information relating to COPD and a very close-knit support group, the members of which keep each other informed of the latest developments in the field. It is a nonprofit association, completely self-supported and accepting no monetary contributions or exclusive affiliations with other entities that might compromise its integrity. Its major goals are to create awareness of COPD, promote research for a cure, and encourage the cessation of smoking.

Increasing Awareness, Research, and Education

COPD is not a popular disease. Many people feel that, as smokers, we did it to ourselves. Many of us, however, started smoking when the dangers of smoking were unknown and when the tobacco companies were putting additive additives in cigarettes. Remember that COPD is a disease that may not manifest itself for 35 years. Therefore, public awareness of COPD needs to be expanded. I have been speaking to various groups at support meetings and at Better Breather clubs, and I am amazed at the lack of knowledge expressed by patients who have had this disease for a long time. Their thirst for basic knowledge is unbelievable.

I also have been in Washington, DC, and have spoken to congressional leaders to try to get increased funding for the National Institutes of Health and resultantly to the Heart, Lung, and Blood Institute for further research into COPD. The lack of knowledge that many congressmen have regarding COPD and the lack of research currently being done is shocking. There are some research programs being conducted, but I feel that more can be done with proper funding.

Most new COPD patients do not know that COPD is the fourth largest cause of death and the second most disabling disease in the United States. The medical community must make these facts known to newly diagnosed patients in order to convince them to take charge of their lives and take better care of themselves. Simply telling them that they have COPD and to stop smoking is not sufficient. Sometimes it is necessary to go to extremes to get someone's attention.

Information on simple breathing techniques and "daily living" suggestions can improve the quality of life for a COPD patient and should be provided. It is also apparent that primary care physicians are not referring patients to pulmonologists in a timely manner. Testing is not being done early enough to determine the severity and progression of the patients' condition. There must be psychological counseling, dietary instructions, and disease progression education during the early stages in an effort to slow down the progression of COPD.

Many of the objectives I have outlined can be accomplished through pulmonary rehabilitation. Some physicians do not advocate this therapy. I suppose some of the objections may be related to cost; in addition, patients may not discipline themselves to continue the exercise and use the knowledge they obtain. Some physicians do not feel that pulmonary rehabilitation will prolong the life of a COPD patient. I can only say to them: "I have this disease. You do not. I am living proof that it works." Rehabilitation may not prolong my life one additional day, but it certainly has given me a quality of life that I never expected to have a few short years ago.

I have found respiratory therapists to be a close and caring community, and they can be tremendous resources for primary care physicians and pulmonologists. However, they are not being utilized enough, nor are there enough educational pulmonary rehabilitation programs being developed. Encouraging COPD patients to join and participate in a pulmonary support group can also be a very useful vehicle in getting across some education and daily living tips.

Physicians need to give their patients these opportunities.

14

Nontraditional Approaches to COPD

Hormoz Ashtyani, MD, and Kristin Fless, MD

Chronic obstructive pulmonary disease (COPD) continues to be a growing health concern, affecting 14 million people or approximately 5% of the US population (American Lung Assn 1987). This disorder is responsible for 90,000 deaths per year, placing it fifth among the leading causes of mortality. COPD is a disabling lung disease with diverse etiologies causing dysfunction of the airways and increased lung volume. Patients with COPD suffer from a disabling shortness of breath, impairing the quality of their life. Routine treatment consists of polypharmacy, which underscores the difficulties the physician encounters treating the many symptoms and morbidities associated with COPD. The standard approach to treatment has focused on the reduction of inflammation and spasm of the airways and improvement of oxygenation. These treatments also may affect mucous production, respiratory muscle function, or control of breathing, leading to secondary gains associated with traditional treatment options. The widespread prevalence of this illness and its impact on a patient's quality of life lead to consideration of other treatment options beyond the traditional medical approach to COPD and whether these should become a part of patient care. The impact of pulmonary rehabilitation, nutritional therapy, pharmacotherapy for breathlessness, noninvasive ventilatory support, and sleep improvement were evaluated as adjunctive treatments of COPD.

Pulmonary Rehabilitation

Pulmonary rehabilitation programs are emerging as a growing treatment option for patients with COPD. These programs often combine exercise training, education, breathing retraining, and social support. Patients are taught how to use abdominal and pursed-lip breathing to improve the mechanics of respiration. These maneuvers have been shown to increase tidal volume, decrease respiratory rate and decrease the oxygen ventilation equivalent (V_E/V_{O_2}) at rest and with exercise (Meuller et al 1970). Despite the improvement in ventilation demonstrated in an early study by Mueller et al, there was no change in gas exchange and not all subjects experienced relief of shortness of breath with pursed-lip breathing. Cambach et al (1997), in a randomized controlled trial with a crossover design, demonstrated an improvement in exercise tolerance and quality of life as measured by the Chronic Respiratory Disease Questionnaire after completion of a pulmonary rehabilitation program. Interestingly, in this study, improvement in the quality of life did not correlate with increased exercise tolerance, suggesting that some other element of comprehensive pulmonary rehabilitation in addition to exercise training was beneficial.

Nutritional Therapy

Much research has been done investigating the importance of nutritional status for patients with COPD. Poor nutrition may contribute to decreased production of surfactant and increase susceptibility to infection. As many as 30% to 50% of COPD patients have reduced muscle mass (Mannix 1999). Reduced muscle mass has been shown to account for decreased aerobic capacity and exercise tolerance (Palange 1995). These patients also demonstrate an increased resting energy expenditure that has been ascribed to the increased work of breathing (Mannix 1999). This has led researchers to investigate the role of nutritional programs for the adjunctive treatment of COPD. Unfortunately, there is scarce information about the role of outpatient nutritional therapy. A small study that enrolled 12 patients in a dietitian-supervised program for 4 months demonstrated very little success, with a mean weight gain of 0.3 kg by the 9 subjects completing the study (Sridhar 1994). This poor outcome certainly suggests that these programs as they are currently implemented will not preserve muscle mass. To compound the issue, evidence suggests that what little lean body mass is present in COPD patients is dysfunctional (Kutsuzawa 1995, Serres 1998). There appears to be a derangement of oxidative metabolism that is present in the muscles of patients with COPD that is independent of nutritional status. It is possible that the causes of decreased muscle mass as well as the treatment are multifactorial.

Nutritional programs are a tempting treatment option and are unlikely to adversely affect patients; however, more studies demonstrating the best way to supplement the care of patients with outpatient programs are needed before they can be recommended as an effective treatment option.

Pharmaceutical Treatment of Breathlessness

Medications to treat the symptom of breathlessness, as well as medications hypothesized to stimulate breathing, have been investigated. Progesterone and acetazolamide have been used to stimulate breathing. Although these medications are often used for patients with hypercapnic respiratory failure, the evidence suggests that COPD patients with hypercapnea have an increased central respiratory drive, but are unable to ventilate well due to neuromechanical derangements (Montes de Oca and Celli 1998).

Breathlessness and the anxiety that occurs with it are symptoms that enfeeble patients with COPD and impair their quality of life and therefore would seem to be good targets for effective pharmaceutical treatment. Although these agents are used clinically for this purpose, the evidence to support their use in chronic COPD is minimal. Poole et al (1998) evaluated the effect of sustained released morphine on quality of life and breathlessness in COPD patients. No improvement was found in quality of life or breathlessness, and the 6-minute walking distance with morphine decreased. Again, this may be limited to a small sample size. Woodcock et al (1981) found that dihydrocodeine reduced breathlessness, improved exercise tolerance, and reduced ventilation and oxygen consumption at rest. Pharmaceutical treatment for the relief of dyspnea and anxiety remains an attractive option.

Noninvasive Ventilatory Support

Noninvasive ventilation (NIV) is gaining widespread acceptance as a treatment option for patients with an exacerbation of COPD. It is used alone to reduce the need for intubation and mechanical ventilation and to bridge the transition from mechanical ventilation to spontaneous ventilation (Nava 1998, Marino 1991). The use of NIV in the stable COPD patient is still awaiting widespread acceptance. Noninvasive ventilation can be used to improve blood gases, decrease work of breathing, alleviate breathlessness, and reduce muscle fatigue. Jones et al (1998) prospectively studied 11 patients with severe stable COPD with hypercapnea on NIV at home for 2 years and found that physician and hospital visits were reduced by half, body mass index did not change, and arterial blood gases improved.

Despite the increased acceptance of NIV by physicians, its use is limited by patient compliance. In the authors' experience at Hackensack University Medical Center, there were 1054 inpatient days of NIV by 264 patients. Compliance for NIV in such patients is currently being evaluated; however, the clinical impression is that compliance is poor. How to make it work? It is proposed that interaction between a specially trained staff on a dedicated NIV unit would significantly improve compliance. Approximately 500 patients per year initiate NIV in the sleep lab at the Institute for Sleep Wake Disorders at Hackensack University Medical Center. Although the data on compliance with NIV are being evaluated, as previously mentioned, staff that can monitor and modify the ventilation and the delivery device would clinically improve the compliance with NIV. A monitored setting would also eliminate the fear of respiratory depression that may inhibit the use of anxiolytics or narcotics in these patients.

Recognition of Impaired Sleep in COPD

Improving sleep-related respiratory disturbances in patients with COPD remains a tangible goal. Normal physiologic changes that occur in sleep such as mild oxygen desaturation, increased upper airway resistance, and the muscle paralysis that occurs with REM sleep exacerbate the respiratory difficulties in the patient who already has perturbed respiratory mechanics and hypoxia. COPD patients may experience apnea and hypopnea in REM sleep if they depend upon accessory muscle use to maintain ventilation. Patients who are borderline hypoxemic and live on the steep part of the oxyhemoglobin/saturation curve may experience significant hypoxia during the normal mild oxygen desaturation that occurs with sleep. We have found that COPD patients as a group have a higher incidence of sleep apnea than the general population. The older age group of patients with COPD, as well as the metabolic derangements that they experience, may contribute to a higher incidence of periodic limb movements in sleep. Because of respiratory disturbances, the maintenance of sleep is poor. Patients should be questioned on the quality of their sleep. They should be asked if they feel refreshed on awakening, or if they experience tiredness during the day. A history should include whether there is evidence of periodic limb movements in sleep, snoring, or other disturbances. Noninvasive ventilation during sleep in COPD patients has been shown to improve sleep efficiency (Krachman 1997). Sleep laboratory monitoring can facilitate the safe use of medications to improve sleep maintenance. Improving the quality of sleep can improve quality of life. A pulmonary and sleep laboratory cooperative effort may be very beneficial in the diagnosis and treatment of nocturnal disorders in COPD patients.

Clearly no one adjunctive treatment for COPD will provide enough benefit to recommend it above all others. There has been increased sensitivity by the medical community to the importance of treating chronic pain; it is proposed that living with the symptom of breathlessness for COPD patients is analogous to living with chronic pain. Aggressive treatment of breathlessness should be the primary goal of COPD treatment. The physician should strive to increase survival if possible and improve the quality of life for patients with chronic lung disease. Several modes of treatment for COPD appear promising, but further investigation of efficacy is pending. Currently the most favorable treatment of COPD involves a multidisciplinary approach, using the above treatment strategies, individualized for each patient.

References

American Lung Association. 1987. *Statistical Compendium on Adult Lung Disease.* New York.

Cambach, W, RV Chadwick-Straver, RC Wagenaar et al. 1997. The effects of a community based pulmonary rehabilitation programme on exercise tolerance and quality of life: a randomized controlled trial. *Eur Respir J.* 10(1):104-113.

Jones, SE, S Packham, M Hebden, and AP Smith. 1998. Domiciliary nocturnal intermittent positive pressure ventilation in patients with respiratory failure due to severe COPD: long-term follow up and effect on survival. *Thorax.* 53(6):495-498.

Krachman, SL, AJ Quaranta, TJ Berger, and CJ Criner. 1997. Effects of non-invasive positive pressure ventilation on gas exchange and sleep in COPD patients. *Chest.* 112(3):623-628.

Kutsuzawa, T, S Shioya, D Kurita et al. 1995. Muscle energy metabolism and nutritional status in patients with chronic obstructive pulmonary disease: a 31P magnetic resonance study. *Am J Resp Crit Care Med.* 152(2):647-652.

Mannix, ET, F Manfredi, and MO Farber. 1999. Elevated O_2 cost of ventilation contributes to tissue wasting in COPD. *Chest.* 115(3):708-713.

Marino, W. 1991. Intermittent volume cycled mechanical ventilation via nasal mask in patients with respiratory failure due to COPD. *Chest.* 99(3):681-684.

Meuller, RE, TL Petty, and GF Filley. 1970. Ventilation and arterial blood gas changes induced by pursed lips breathing. *J Applied Physiology.* 28(6):784-789.

Montes de Oca, M and BR Celli. 1998. Mouth occlusion pressure, CO_2 response and hypercapnea in severe chronic obstructive pulmonary disease. *Eur Respir J.* 12:66-67.

Nava, S, N Ambrosino, E Clini et al. 1998. Non-invasive mechanical ventilation in the weaning of patients with respiratory failure due to chronic obstructive pulmonary disease: a randomized, controlled trial. *Annals Int Med.* 128(9):721-728.

Palange, P, S Forte, A Felli et al. 1995. Nutritional state and exercise tolerance in patients with COPD. *Chest.* 107(5):1206-12.

Poole, PJ, AG Veale, and PN Black. 1998. The effect of sustained release morphine on breathlessness and quality of life in severe chronic obstructive pulmonary disease. *Am J Resp Crit Care Med.* 157(6 pt 1):1877-1880.

Serres, I, M Hayot, C Prefaut, and J Mercier. 1998. Skeletal muscle abnormalities in patients with COPD: contribution to exercise intolerance. *Med and Sci in Sports & Exercise.* 30(7):1019-1027.

Sridhar, MK, A Galloway, ME Lean, and SW Banham. 1994. An out-patient nutritional supplementation programme in COPD patients. *Eur Respir J.* 7(4):720-724.

Woodcock, AA, ER Gross, A Gellert et al. 1981. Effects of dihydrocodeine, alcohol, and caffeine on breathlessness and exercise tolerance in patients with chronic obstructive pulmonary disease. *New Eng J Med.* 305(27):1611-1616.

15

Mind-Body Connection and COPD

Sreedhar Nair, MD

Most people are led to believe that this is a material world, that we are what we have achieved and what we possess. But, scientifically, it is a mental world, because we see the world through the prism of the mind—that consciousness that is the animating force of life, and not the ego, which is only an internal reference point. In the words of Anais Nin, "We don't see things as they are; we see things as we are"(1969).

The impact of the mind and the emotions on body functions has been demonstrated by many scientists for more than a century. Deep emotions, like sorrow and anger, can produce, as well as aggravate, illness; other emotions, such as happiness and hope, can prevent and improve the same illnesses. As the sorrow and suffering of illness help patients better understand the basic realities and relationships of their lives, many change their lifestyles. Those who do, survive longer and live happier lives. Why?

In order to understand the mind-body interaction, we should look at the nature of a whole person. It consists of the body, the intellect, emotions and relationships, and the deep consciousness, which we call the soul, from which springs all spirituality.

The Body

Good nutrition, sleep, and relaxation—or the lack of them—all greatly affect our sense of well-being. A diet that is largely vegetarian and high-fiber has the least adverse impact on our bodies. In addition, diet, drugs, and emotions affect sleep, and without adequate sleep, the body simply wears out. This is especially true for patients with chronic obstructive pulmonary disease (COPD) and emphysema. Many body functions, such as shortness of breath and muscle spasms, can be altered and improved by relaxation techniques, meditation, and prayer.

It is also important to realize that all matter has an intrinsic resonance— be it our bodies with their cells, molecules, and atoms or the external world itself. When the intrinsic resonance of our bodies is in harmony with nature and the external forces of life, we feel happy, invigorated, and well. In many disease states, such as asthma and emphysema, there is a disharmony in the intrinsic resonance. Many of these malfunctions can be demonstrated and observed in certain centers of the midbrain by magnetic resonance imaging and other techniques. Moreover, neuroscientists in the Netherlands have found that producing a chantlike sound that matches the resonance of an illness can improve or eliminate symptoms of that disease. Yogic breathing exercises with chanting of mantras have been known to improve shortness of breath, a predominant symptom of COPD and emphysema, but much more research must still be done in this area.

The Intellect

The 20th century has been an age of science, of discovery and quantum leaps in man's knowledge of our material world. But these advances have not answered the questions that most of us have regarding what life is all about: Why are we on this earth? How did we come to be? Where will we be going ultimately? In the last few years, physicists and astronomers have converged with philosophers as they ask these eternal questions, having reached the brink of knowledge and witnessed the timelessness and vastness of space that no equation can solve. We as physicians should also ask these questions, because we are the ones who see the suffering and death, the arbitrariness of life.

These questions have challenged mankind from its beginning. We know that they cannot be answered by scientific inquiry but only by belief systems and spiritual forces immeasurable by any meter or oscilloscope. The intellect likes to be objective, rational, and scientific, requiring proof of everything. It is limited and possessive; it divides and encapsulates us. But the spirit reaches out to the rest of humanity and connects us with the universe. As physicians and caregivers we need to understand that, although it is the intellect and its technology that cures, it is the spiritual aspect of the caregiver and the patient that bonds them together and heals.

Emotions and Relationships

Literature shows that an optimistic approach to life, with laughter and hope, is associated with increased survival, and that depression, anger, fear, and interpersonal conflicts reduce the life span. Very often, fear dominates our lives: fear of losing, fear of illness, fear of dying. The root cause of fear is duality: I versus you. We try to possess more and more objects, to no avail; otherwise, the richest men would be the happiest. We build boundaries and separate ourselves from the rest of the world. We separate ourselves from others by religion, race, ethnicity, and country, and we are prepared to kill each other over these. That is why, during most of history, mankind has been consumed by violence and war. If, instead, we take a larger view, then we should be able to look at life without the fear of dying because dying is absolutely safe. Near-death experiences of many people have taught us that. In many cultures death is a celebration of the end of a rich and fulfilling life.

Spirituality

One of the most important areas of research in the mind-body connection is that of spirituality and religion and their influence on illness. Few of us have the time or desire to get in touch with our inner consciousness, which is essentially the hallmark of all humanity. It is the same consciousness that connects us with the rest of the universe and is part of the cosmic force that binds all living things together. Patients suffering from emphysema and COPD should start on a program of renovation of their psyches. In other words, they should seek self-awareness and self-knowledge, and lead a life of what the Buddhists call "mindfulness," or mindful living (Nhat 1992). Patients should experience the joys of contributing to the welfare of others and helping those less fortunate. They must get in touch with themselves and find their center and look at the illness, not as an isolated phenomenon, but rather as part of the whole world of suffering. Nature, meditation, prayer, and the arts can help patients get in touch with themselves and with the cosmic world and all its resonance and radiance.

Nature, with its infinite beauty, is all around us and we yearn to be part of it. That is why we choose to vacation in places of great natural splendor. We do not go to Hoboken for a honeymoon; we go to Bermuda, Sedona, Hawaii, and the national parks. We go to Niagara Falls. Standing there with our ears to the thundering water and our eyes to the luminous mist, we suddenly see a rainbow and understand what Byron meant when he wrote, "Who hath not felt the might, the majesty of loveliness?" We become part of the mystery and wonder around us. Psychologists call this "peak experience," James Joyce called it epiphany, and Joseph Campbell called it the rapture of being alive.

Patients who cannot solve deep problems are often advised to go to the seashore and gaze at the setting sun and then, as darkness falls, at the moon and the vastness of the sky and the stars as they begin to shine. Viewing themselves against the backdrop of the immensity of space tends to make their problems become smaller, less important. They realize that their life span on this planet is very short in comparison. This technique is called the "sky watch program," which has benefited people, even children, with chronic diseases and depression.

All these peak experiences add to personal growth, like rungs on a ladder that take us higher and higher in the evolutionary spiral of spirituality and let us partake in something greater than the human dimension. We become harmonious with the rhythms of nature, and there is a graceful unfolding of our lives that leads to an inner transformation, peace, and creative energy.

Prayer and meditation also lead us to a higher spirituality. When we pray, we speak to our God; when we meditate, we speak to our own souls. To meditate, we must look within ourselves and, with the inner eye, see our thoughts go by. The mind has been described as a restless monkey who got drunk and was stung by a bee. As we watch our thoughts go by, they will become less and less frequent. The technique lies in focusing on the gap between thoughts where one thought ends and the other begins. As we try to widen this gap, we will look down and see, and become aware of, our inner consciousness. This will be a truly mystical experience, helping us to see the oneness of all life and the interrelatedness of all living things.

We must pour out our love—to children, grandchildren, other loved ones, pets—and see how much the giving and receiving of love can do for us. When we experience that love, or when we listen to our favorite music or look at a great painting at the art museum or read our favorite book, we have a feeling that time stops, and we are aware that we are part of eternity. If we live intensely in the present, from moment to moment in a mindful fashion, we will enjoy life without fear. Even though life may seem to be full of sadness and suffering, we'll be able (as Joseph Campbell once paraphrased a Buddhist saying) "to participate joyously in the sorrows of life."

References

Nhat, HT. 1992. *Peace Is Every Step: the Path of Mindfulness in Everyday Life.* New York, NY: Bantam Books.

Nin, A. 1969. *The Diary of Anais Nin, 1939-1944.* New York, NY: Harcourt Brace and World.

16

Methods for Getting Physicians to Accept Self-Help Groups

Joseph F. Fennelly, MD

The perspective in the following material is that of a self-help group member. Regardless of the extent of dysfunction, the social support, coping skills, and competence provided by membership in a self-help group can significantly reduce stress and lessen constitutional vulnerabilities. The help provided by such groups and their members is too broad to be discussed here, so I will dwell on a few high points that may be of interest to physicians.

Self-Help Group Principles and Mechanisms

Self-help group members share a number of principles that guide their activities in ways that may be supportive of the medical care provided by physicians. These include the helper therapy principle, a belief that one of the best ways members can help themselves is through helping others. Members also act as positive role models ("If I can do it, you can"), are accessible at almost any time (no office hour limitations), provide a sense of normalcy even in the case of severely stigmatizing conditions, and offer strategies and support to cope with and, if possible, prevent the condition.

The opportunities provided by self-help groups for service and altruism give members meaning and a sense of empowerment. In addition, self-help groups frequently furnish:

- *Unique expertise.* Self-help groups are unique resources because of the members' personal experience with the condition.
- *Sophisticated communication skills.* Self-help groups are increasingly in the forefront of technology use, employing computers, the Internet, and e-mail to facilitate communication among members and with health care systems and professionals. Groups related to chronic obstructive pulmonary disease (COPD), with members that may have restricted mobility, sometimes provide training on using these modalities.
- *Feedback and feed-forward loop.* Physicians and self-help group members educate and support one another.

Establishing a Relationship With Physicians

Currently, medical education emphasizes technological answers and focuses on teaching physicians how to "fix what needs fixing." Since modern technology has produced profound changes in physicians' "fixing" skills, the technology itself can overwhelm and blind educators to other ways of knowing. Magic bullets help us in the war against some diseases, but to the extent that we are often diverted from our inability to address many other diseases and chronic conditions.

The majesty of modern health care institutions, awesome temples of healing with august white walls and panoramic windows, makes the Taj Mahal look like a sandcastle. In these hallowed temples, physicians do modern magic: change genes, replace hearts, and send children to school on permanent respirators. People become part human, part technology.

The movie "The Doctor" provides an example of how powerful the physician and modern science have become in society. William Hurt plays a heart transplant surgeon, a supremely confident, if not arrogant, physician, who becomes ill himself. Prior to his illness, the character defined compassion as getting in out of the belly as fast as possible. In one scene, he strides into a room where a minister is sitting beside a patient in traction for injuries sustained from a suicide attempt. When the minister asks if he is in the way, the surgeon simply stands silently, conveying the impression that the real help has arrived. As the minister scurries out, the patient continues to express his dismay about his suicide attempt to the surgeon, who flippantly replies in a monotone, "If you want to commit suicide, try golf." Until he becomes ill and learns the value of peer support, the surgeon feels that his technical skills are all that he needs.

This character exemplifies those physicians who perceive that they can perform the miracles previously attributed to holy figures, obviating the need for communities of faith as part of health and healing. Our medicalized society does not value intuition, and the language of physicians leaves little room for uncertainty and ambiguity or for expressing and understanding subjective pain and suffering. To help people with advanced COPD, where do physicians learn, through passionate, poignant expression, what it means to feel starved for oxygen, to never get a full breath? The answer, of course, is from self-help groups, which give patients the voice to talk poetically about the horror of "drowning in an ocean of air" and the courage to speak up to the "MDeities."

Access Routes to Self-Help Groups

Of the many ways for physicians to access the assistance available through self-help groups, the most readily available may be following the examples of physicians who have responded to their own patients' needs. As indicated above, the experience of people with a particular disease or condition gives them unique expertise that physicians can tap into. Physicians such as "Dr. Bob," who helped "Bill" start Alcoholics Anonymous, and former Surgeon General C. Everett Koop, MD, serve as invaluable role models. In 1987, Dr. Koop developed a national agenda for recognizing and utilizing the public health contributions of self-help groups by sponsoring the Surgeon General's Workshop on Self-Help and Public Health and supporting publication of the workshop proceedings. Dr. Koop has written and spoken widely about his experiences as a medical practitioner and as an organizer and member of self-help groups, and about what he learned of the importance of self-help groups in assisting their members in dealing with problems, stress, hardship, and pain.

My own experiences have taught me similar lessons. Thirty years ago, after performing pulmonary rehabilitation in my office, I started the first hospital-based cardiac rehabilitation program. I persuaded other physicians to allow their patients to participate in the program by rewording the standing orders to require a signature if the physician did not want the patient rehabilitated. In the same standing order, I included a sentence requesting physicians to sign if they objected to their patients being visited by heart attack survivors from occupations similar to that of the patients. Few physicians signed.

When asked about the most positive experience they had in the hospital during rehabilitation for their heart attack, patients invariably responded that it was the self-help group member from their own occupation (police officer, firefighter, housewife, airline pilot, etc.) who volunteered, on their own time, to use their survivor expertise to help patients cope with the multiple ramifications of their condition.

Selective Use of Self-Help Resources

I refer patients and their family members to different self-help groups for different conditions. As with referrals and consultants, physicians need to know something about the philosophies of different groups and how they operate. Whenever I cannot match family members suffering a loss or tragedy with a self-help group, I refer them to a trustworthy source, the American Self-Help Clearinghouse, 1-800-FOR-MASH (Mutual Aid Self-Help). Every medical student, every resident, and every practicing physician should know this number by heart.

Helping physicians fit self-help group resources into the prevailing system can be this simple and this subtle. Physicians are beginning to welcome help in empowering their patients, as we hear more and more about patient-centered care and patient autonomy. Changing health care systems, with the emphasis on managed-care economics, rapid discharge, and a more holistic "team" approach (as reflected by new standards from the Joint Commission on Accreditation of Healthcare Organizations), increase the attractiveness of self-help groups as partners in health care. More and more hospitals are hosting self-help groups, and more and more staff are referring patients to group support not provided by the institution. Physician flow sheets for patients' care can even include self-help groups, whether involved in curative or palliative care.

COPD, by its very nature, poses additional challenges. Cancer, which is more time-predictable, provides some self-help models, but COPD needs a more inclusive approach. And we as physicians need to change the rituals of medicine to embrace cultural differences, especially in life-threatening illnesses, such as advanced COPD. Toward this end, the AMA's *1999 Cultural Competence Compendium*, edited by Hannah Hedrick, PhD, provides resources on the "culture" of end-of-life care and on self-help groups, which can assist physicians wishing to increase their knowledge about, or develop a relationship with, self-help groups.

Physicians can also assume helpful roles in self-help groups, as long as they understand that the leadership of autonomous groups comes from within the groups and is not subject to professional control. For example, physicians can encourage groups to be even more inclusive in their development of a sense of community. As physicians participate in this process of empowerment provided by self-help groups, they will reap personal and professional benefits that will help the self-help movement increase geometrically. Although this may appear to require a drastic paradigm shift in modeling and education, it is encouraging to note that much progress has already been made, as evidenced by the presentations at the 1999 Symposium on Advanced Chronic Obstructive Pulmonary Disease, hosted by The American Institute of Life-Threatening Illness and Loss. We all owe a tremendous debt of gratitude to The American Institute's president, Dr. Austin Kutscher, a pioneer not only in end-of-life care, but also in the bringing together of members of various medical and related professions with patients and their families to identify and satisfy unmet needs.

As a result of Dr. Kutscher's leadership, professionals and grassroots self-help groups are moving forward together to provide awareness of the unrelenting symptoms of COPD, to emphasize the importance of relieving caregiver burden, to provide tools for dealing with anger, to develop nicotine-addiction awareness programs, and to promote the use of self-help groups as resources. I encourage physicians to join these and other initiatives designed to change the belief systems that prevent health care professionals from understanding and embracing self-help groups. As we do so, we not only help our patients, we help ourselves.

Part II

Palliative Care
and
End-of-Life Issues

17

Controlling COPD Symptoms

Helen M. Sorenson, RRT

*The tragedy of old age is not that each of us must grow old and die,
but that the process of doing so has been made unnecessarily and at times
excruciatingly painful, humiliating, debilitating and isolating.*
—Robert Butler

Chronic obstructive pulmonary disease (COPD), a slowly disabling and progressively destructive disease that is often fatal, is now the fourth leading cause of death in the United States (Scanlan et al 1999). While mortality rates from other cardiac and cerebrovascular disease have declined, the incidence of COPD-related death has increased, likely paralleling smoking trends. Between 1980 and 1995, there was a 58.7% increase in the death rate from COPD, per 100,000 population (US Bureau of the Census 1998).

By definition, the chronic nature of COPD implies persistence of the condition over a long period of time. The 2 diseases most commonly associated with COPD are chronic bronchitis and emphysema. Chronic bronchitis, without any comorbid conditions, is treatable and reversible. Emphysema is manageable. Some newer forms of therapy are available on a limited basis. Lung transplantation, lung volume reduction surgery, and intravenous augmentation with a purified protein preparation of alpha 1-antitrypsin from human blood donors may buy the patient a few extra years. Defined in anatomical terms, however, emphysema is permanent and irreversible.

End-stage COPD is characterized either by a slowly developing or a rapidly advancing exacerbation. COPD patients, on the continuum of psychological adjustment, range anywhere between eternal optimism and abject pessimism. The optimists do not want to discuss end-of-life issues. Many have been brought back from near death before and see exacerbations as serious but not life ending. Pessimists often say that they do not care how and when they die, and frequently continue to smoke. Those COPD patients in the middle of the spectrum are concerned with their disease management/outcome, but the chronic nature of the condition can give them a false sense of longevity. While most COPD patients have definite opinions on end-of-life care, they often wait too long to express their wishes. When exacerbations lead to respiratory failure, mechanical ventilation is indicated. The decision not to intubate will most likely result in death. Once it has been determined that heroic measures will not be implemented, the focus needs to center on the control of symptoms and palliative care.

Palliative Care

According to Ahmedzai (1998) in the *Oxford Textbook of Palliative Medicine*, there are 4 general principles of palliation:

1. Determine and treat the underlying cause of symptoms, whenever possible and reasonable for the patient.
2. Relieve symptoms without adding new problems through, for example, side effects, drug interactions, social, or financial burden.
3. Consider whether the treatment will be worthwhile for the patient and family, weighing such factors as prognosis, adverse effects, and social and financial cost.
4. Discuss reasonable treatment options, including "no intervention," with the patient and family, allowing them, as much as is possible, to make the final decision.

Compassionate treatment to the dying must be the ultimate goal. However, successful relief of symptoms that cause undue pain and suffering remains a challenge. Many articles about palliative care appear in medical journals, and the hospice movement has championed the field of palliative medicine for patients with cancer, AIDS, and intractable pain. Hospice care for patients with COPD, however, has generally not been available in the past (Skolnick 1998) and information on palliative care for such patients is also limited.

COPD Symptoms

A study reported in the *Annals of Internal Medicine* (Lynn et al 1997) explored how family members or surrogate decisionmakers perceived the dying process of older patients. The rate of severe symptoms perceived 3 days prior to death of patients with COPD were severe dyspnea–91%, severe pain–34%, and severe confusion–17%. Other commonly observed symptoms in the end stages of COPD were: cough, depression, anxiety, and a syndrome known as anorexia/cachexia.

Dyspnea

Labored or difficult breathing seems to be the most common symptom in end-stage COPD. Dyspnea can result from inadequate ventilation, inadequate oxygenation, an acute infection, atelectasis, pulmonary edema, anxiety, or a variety of other disorders. Determination of the cause, if possible, should drive the symptom management. As with all palliative care, the level of desired intervention may be the determining factor in choice of therapy. (See Table 1.)

Table 1—Control of Dyspnea

Possible Causes	Suggested Interventions
Inadequate ventilation; inadequate oxygenation	Low-flow oxygen, pursed-lip breathing, high Fowler's position, room fan, nebulized opioids, bronchodilators, corticosteroids
Acute infection	Antibiotic therapy*
Atelectasis, pneumothorax, pleural effusion	Low-flow oxygen. Treat as indicated, considering principles of palliation [may include hyperinflation therapy (CPAP, IBBP, IS), chest tube insertion, thoracentesis]*
Pulmonary edema	Low-flow oxygen, diuretics, morphine sulfate, cardiac glycosides*
Anxiety	Low-flow oxygen, pursed-lip breathing, anxiolytic,* room fan

* May or may not be consistent with level of palliative care requested by patient/family.

Every patient, regardless of therapy, should be placed in a comfortable position, using pillows to prop and support. A fan that directs cool air to the patient's face is usually beneficial. Complementary approaches in treating dyspnea, such as relaxation, music therapy, or massage may be advantageous.

Nebulized Opioids

Theoretically, there are a number of reasons why nebulized opioids (opiates) have been advocated in treating dyspnea. According to the *Oxford Textbook of Palliative Medicine*, it has been postulated that opiates

- diminish the ventilatory response to hypoxia, hypercapnia, and exercise
- work centrally, altering the perception of breathlessness
- affect opioid receptors in lung and peripheral tissue to modify the sensation of breathlessness
- relieve dyspnea by indirectly exerting vasodilator action, reducing workload on the heart.

Studies examining the benefits of morphine in treating breathlessness have not all been favorable. A comparison of sustained-release morphine and a placebo on breathlessness in patients with severe COPD demonstrated no measurable difference (Poole et al 1997). This study also showed no significant change in oxygen saturation at rest in patients treated with sustained-release morphine. A different study revealed that in humans, the magnitude of change in ventilation and the sensitivity of the hypercapnic drive were not related to plasma morphine concentrations (Riggs 1978). Two additional studies focusing more on the effect that nebulized morphine had on exercise tolerance revealed little to no significant change between the opioid and the placebo (Beauford et al 1993; Masood et al 1995).

In theory, nebulized opioid administration provides a fast, effective route of administration, reduced systemic side effects, and the ability to administer the drug "as needed." In reality, respiratory therapists across the country are administering nebulized morphine, dilaudid, and fentanyl for the management of dyspnea and intractable cough in terminal COPD patients. Nebulized morphine has been known in some instances, however, to cause bronchial spasm secondary to histamine release. If necessary, albuterol can be administered to treat the bronchospasm. Some institutions choose to nebulize dilaudid or fentanyl, as neither has been shown to trigger an airway reaction. Even though multiple sites have reported favorable results in relieving breathlessness with nebulized opioids, this remains an area where controlled research is greatly needed. To date, anecdotal testimony to the efficacy of nebulized opioids in treating breathlessness has been more widely available than hard clinical data. A case study extolling the benefits of nebulized morphine was published in *Lancet* in 1993, with the statement, however, that the mechanism of action in relieving dyspnea may yet be unknown (Tooms et al 1993).

Pain

Palliative care focuses on reducing the severity and alleviation of unpleasant symptoms. Pain is a major symptom in the terminal stages of life and is usually associated with actual or potential tissue damage.

A study of family members' perceptions of the dying experience of end-stage patients reveals that at least half of the time, during the last 3 days of life, 34% of patients with COPD experience pain of moderate to extreme severity (Lynn et al 1997). The same study also found that 4 in 10 dying patients had severe pain most of the time. An unfortunate reality is that most physicians in the United States have no formal training in palliative care. As a result, patients at the end of life often suffer from a lack of appropriate pain management (Butler 1999).

Because many patients with COPD also have comorbid conditions, it is reasonable to first assess the nature and location of the pain. A determination should be made as to whether the pain is localized or diffuse. Modified scales of 1 to 10, with "1" being little pain and "10" signifying the most intense pain, will quantify for the caregiver what they are treating. Scales will also, to some extent, help caregivers document both subjectively and objectively the changes affected by therapy.

Anti-inflammatory medications may relieve pain caused by edema of interstitial tissue, necrotizing tissue, or inflammation of mucous or serous membranes. Pain caused by direct damage to nerves may not respond to opioids. There are a number of analgesics available that can effectively reduce or blunt the sensation of pain. For COPD patients, the concern has always been respiratory depression. Narcotics affect the central nervous system and also depress respiration. In an effort to prevent drug-induced respiratory failure and the development of an addiction, effective analgesics are probably underused. Newer evidence, however, indicates these fears may be unfounded. It is known clinically that patients with severe pain who receive large doses of opiates rarely, if ever, demonstrate respiratory depression or an addiction when the doses are titrated properly (O'Brien 1996). The rule of double effect, although not applicable for every patient, is important. Under the rule, an action having two effects, one good and one bad, is permissible under the following conditions:

- The act itself is good or at least morally neutral.
- Only the good effect is intended.
- The good effect is not achieved through the bad effect.
- There is no alternative way to attain the good effect.
- There is a proportionally grave reason for not risking the good effect.

When patients and families are informed and consent to the treatment, the end result can be a very effective alleviation of pain (Quill et al 1997).

Alternative therapies, such as Reiki, massage therapy, music therapy, or even the use of topical analgesics are not often documented in medical texts. When performed on accepting patients, these nontraditional methods can be calming, stress reducing, and pain relieving.

Confusion

A major cause of mental disorientation and confusion in end-stage COPD patients is a lack of adequate oxygen in the blood (hypoxemia), which results in low oxygen at the tissue level (hypoxia). Treatment with low-flow oxygen may alleviate the symptoms. There comes a time in palliative care, however, when delivery of a high fraction of inspired oxygen to maintain adequate saturation of hemoglobin becomes pointless. Some would even question the use of monitoring devices in palliative care.

If low-flow oxygen does not decrease a patient's confusion, the medications being delivered for possible side effects or drug-drug interactions should be examined. If the confusion appears related to depression, therapy to stimulate or engage the patient may be beneficial. Pet therapy and/or music therapies are alternatives that should not be discounted.

Cough

Generally, a cough that forcefully expels air from the lungs will also expel secretions. Clearing the airways reduces airway resistance and decreases the work of breathing. Respiratory care practitioners spend a great deal of time coaching their patients to cough. When a cough becomes paroxysmal or intractable, however, it exerts too heavy a toll on the patient and should be suppressed. Treatment of coughing is ideally guided by the underlying cause. (See Table 2.)

Table 2—Control of Cough

Possible Causes	Suggested Interventions
Infection	Antibiotics*
Drug-induced (eg, ACE inhibitor)	Stop the drug; replace with another class
Reflux	Position patient with head elevated
Aspiration of saliva	Anti-cholinergics,* nebulized local anesthetic to reduce sensation*
Reactive airway disease	Bronchodilators, corticosteroids, antitussives*

* May or may not be consistent with level of palliative care requested by patient/family.

It is important when controlling the cough to not add additional problems more distressing than the cough. For example, if constipation is a problem, avoid antitussives with codeine. If the patient is in heart block or suffers from liver or kidney disease, nebulized lidocaine might be avoided. If using over-the-counter cough syrup, the label should be read carefully. Preparations with expectorants will increase the amount of mucus produced. If a productive cough is the goal, expectorants are effective. If cough suppression is the goal, the patient should be given an antitussive.

Depression

Although sadness is common when death approaches, clinical depression is a more serious condition. According to Peck (1997), the most common cause of depression is helpless anger or rage. Illness can trigger both responses. Most patients with COPD who smoked accept the fact that the decision to smoke was, in large part, responsible for their disease. Many patients, however, harbor anger or rage at the tobacco companies or at their physicians who did not "make them quit."

Depression is also a side effect of many medications. When the cause of depression is biochemical, it may be easy to reverse. When the depression is a result of an affective disorder, however, treatment is more complicated. Palliative care is not aggressive. Psychotherapy or shock therapy would probably not be considered appropriate. Antidepressant drugs, though, might be appropriate in the treatment of profound depression.

Unfinished business may be the causative factor in depression. Helpless anger over the dynamics of a family situation may trigger a depressive state. The feeling of not being able to say or do things as intended can lead to hopelessness. Depression robs patients of the opportunity to "finish business." If depression can be reversed, patients in palliative care may be able to use the time remaining and make the process of dying a little easier.

Anxiety

Mild dysphoria or anxiety is fairly common in the last 3 days of life (Lynn et al 1997). Homeostatic equilibrium of the respiratory system in a COPD patient is tenuous at best. Shortness of breath, for whatever reason, can precipitate an attack of anxiety. The anxiety can in turn cause physiologic changes that increase the rate of metabolism, triggering increased oxygen consumption and reduced oxygen delivery. This contributes to increased shortness of breath and concomitant anxiety. If not interrupted, these decrementally cascading events can be very harmful. Low-flow oxygen therapy would be beneficial. Pursed-lip breathing would reduce panic effectively in compliant patients. The cold facial stimulation afforded by a room fan can reduce breathlessness and diminish the anxiety associated with dyspnea. When severe enough to warrant treatment, the symptoms may also be alleviated by social support or anxiolytics.

Anorexia/Cachexia

The anorexia/cachexia syndrome is more common in terminal cancer patients than in COPD patients, but it is not uncommon in end-stage COPD. Anorexia is a result of diminished appetite. Cachexia, characterized by malnutrition, overall weakness, generalized muscle atrophy, and loss of body mass, is a result of anorexia.

Some patients with COPD, given a limited amount of energy, find that eating is too exhausting. Anecdotal patient comments relate some loss of appetite to low-flow (long-term) oxygen therapy. Dysphagia, dry mouth, mouth sores, hypoxemia, medication side effects, and depression can all cause altered food intake. Deprivation of food, for whatever reason, results in starvation and adds to the level of suffering.

Parenteral nutrition is an option for patients and families to consider, but one that is not always used. Perhaps optimal nutritional management would best be served by gentle encouragement to maintain fluid intake via ice chips, for example, or sips of water. Additionally, any food the patient will consume should be provided, regardless of nutritional value.

Conclusion

Palliative care, terminal care, and acceptance into hospice have been designated as appropriate during the last 6 months of life. Patients with COPD, however, may be fairly stable until the final period of deterioration. Realistically, there may not be time for hospice placement. A clear understanding of the level of medical intervention desired by patients and their families is imperative. If comfort care is the choice, then health care providers who are knowledgeable about and sympathetic to the goals of palliative care can work with patients and families in providing adequate symptom relief. As Robert Twycross (1990), borrowing a quote from Sir William Osler, states: "Palliative care means to cure sometimes, to relieve often, to comfort always."

References

Ahmedzai, S. 1998. Palliation of respiratory symptoms. In *Oxford Textbook of Palliative Medicine*, eds. D Doyle, GWC Hanks, and N McDonald. 2nd ed. Oxford University Press.

Beauford, W, TT Saylor, DW Stansbury, K Avalos, and RW Light. 1993. Effects of nebulized morphine sulfate on the exercise tolerance of the ventilatory limited COPD patient. *Chest*. 104(1):175-178.

Butler, R. 1999. Handbook for mortals. *Geriatrics*. 54(5):3.

———. 1975. *Why Survive? Being Old in America*, 3. New York, NY: Harper and Row.

Lynn, J, J Teno, RS Phillips et al. 1997. Perceptions by family members of the dying experience of older and seriously ill patients. *Ann Int Med*. 126(2):97-105.

Masood, AR, JW Reed, and SHL Thomas. 1995. Lack of effect of inhaled morphine on exercise induced breathlessness in COPD. *Thorax*. 50:629-634.

O'Brien, CP. 1996. Drug addiction and drug abuse. In *Goodman and Gilman's The Pharmalogical Basis of Therapeutics*, eds. AG Goodman, JG Hardman, LE Limbird, PB Molinoff, and RW Rodden. 9th ed. New York, NY: McGraw-Hill Book Co.

Peck, MS. 1997. *Denial of the Soul*. New York, NY: Harmony Books.

Poole, PJ, AG Veale, and PN Black. 1997. The effect of sustained-release morphine on breathlessness and quality of life in severe COPD. *Am J Resp Crit Care Med*. 157:1877-1880.

Quill, TE, R Dresser, and DW Brock. 1997. The rule of double effect: a critique of its role in end-of-life decision making. *New Eng J Med*. 337:1768-1771.

Riggs, JRA. 1978. Ventilatory effects and plasma concentration of morphine in man. *Brit J Anesthesia*. 50:759-765.

Scanlan, CL, RL Wilkins, and JK Stoller. 1999. *Egan's Fundamentals of Respiratory Care*. St. Louis, MO: Mosby, Inc.

Skolnick, AA. 1998. MediCaring project to demonstrate, evaluate innovative end-of-life program for chronically ill. *JAMA*. 279(19):1511-1512.

Tooms, A, A McKenzie, and H Grey. 1993. Nebulized morphine. *Lancet*. 342:1123-1124.

Twycross, R. 1990. Why palliative medicine. Keynote presentation, 6th international hospice institute symposium. Jul 20. Estes Park, CO.

US Bureau of the Census. 1998. *Statistical Abstract of the United States.* 118th ed. Washington, DC.

18

Palliative Care for Sleep and Sleep Disorders in COPD

Barbara Ann Phillips, MD, MSPh, FCCP

Sleep Changes With Age

Several investigators have defined normal changes in sleep that occur with aging (Bliwise 1993, Ancoli-Israel 1997, Miles and Dement 1980). Sleep becomes more fragmented and both arousals and awakenings increase. Both rapid-eye movement (REM) and slow wave sleep decrease. There are increased numbers of sleep stage shifts, indicating difficulty in maintaining states and stages. There are fewer REM/non-REM cycles, and ultimately reduced sleep efficiency (the ratio of time spent sleeping to time spent in bed). Electroencephalographic changes in sleep occur as well, with a reduction in amplitude of slow waves and in the numbers of sleep spindles.

Many older people "phase advance," resulting from a forward shift of the circadian rhythm. Older adults get sleepy earlier than they did when they were younger and have a tendency to wake up earlier. Ancoli-Israel (1997) has demonstrated that this contributes to the common problem of early morning awakening in this age group.

Development of health problems also has an impact on sleep in the elderly. Bliwise (1993) notes that nocturia, headache, gastrointestinal illness, bronchitis, cardiovascular symptoms, diabetes, menopause, osteoarthritis, and medication side effects have all been shown to disrupt sleep in the elderly. He also points out that controversy exists about whether there is actually decreased sleep need with aging; older adults who are healthy tend to get and to need about as much sleep as they did when younger, although it may be distributed differently during the 24-hour period.

Sleep Complaints in the Aged

Sleep complaints are common in the geriatric age group, with more than half of the elderly endorsing a complaint about their sleep quality (Foley et al 1995). The most common complaint is difficulty with maintenance of sleep. In the survey conducted by Foley and colleagues, reports of poor sleep correlated strongly both with health complaints and with depressive symptoms. Rediehs and colleagues (1990) point out that although women are more likely to complain of sleep difficulty than are men, their sleep may actually be better preserved than that of their male counterparts. Interestingly, daytime napping correlates weakly with increased mortality, perhaps because it is a marker for significant nocturnal sleep disturbance (Foley et al).

Humans experience impaired mood, reduced vigilance, deterioration of memory, and an increased risk of automobile accidents with sleep restriction (Friedman et al 1973, Leighton and Livingston 1983, Wilkinson 1963, Martin S et al 1996, Marcus and Loughlin 1996). Sleep deprivation has also been shown to increase the collapsibility of the upper airway (Series et al 1994) and reduce respiratory drive (Cooper and Phillips 1982). Sleep loss also impairs performance on pulmonary function testing, both in healthy older humans (Phillips et al 1989) and in older patients with chronic obstructive pulmonary disease (COPD) (Phillips et al 1987). It is tempting to postulate that the sleep changes that almost invariably accompany aging contribute to the increased prevalence of sleep-disordered breathing (SDB) in this group.

Effects of Sleep on Breathing

Breathing deteriorates during sleep for most humans. Brown (1998) provides an excellent review of this topic. There are multiple causes for breathing problems during sleep, including reduced respiratory drive, increased upper airway resistance, loss of muscle tone, ventilation-perfusion (V/Q) mismatch, and reduced functional residual capacity (FRC). Respiratory impairment during sleep is generally more extreme during REM sleep than during non-REM sleep. REM sleep is associated with an upper motor neuron paralysis that causes loss of muscle tone throughout the body. Only the diaphragm, extraocular muscles, and muscles of the middle ear are spared.

Ventilatory response to both hypoxemia and hypercarbia has been shown to decline during sleep, particularly during REM sleep (Douglas et al 1982). Thus, humans "tolerate" both lower oxygen tensions and higher carbon dioxide tensions more during sleep than while awake.

Patency of the upper airway is maintained by upper airway pharyngeal dilator muscles. Compared with wakefulness, these muscles have reduced tone (eg, are more flaccid) during non-REM sleep, and have marked atonia in REM sleep. Several investigators (White et al 1995, Meurice et al 1995) have demonstrated that both normal individuals and patients with COPD experience increased upper airway resistance as a result of the reduction in activity of the pharyngeal dilator muscles that accompanies sleep. Further, the accessory muscles of respiration, including the scalenes, intercostal, sternomastoids, and abdominal wall muscles, can no longer contribute to ventilation during REM sleep. Patients with COPD are particularly dependent on these accessory muscles. Johnson and Remmers (1984) demonstrated significant dropout of muscle tone in the scalene and sternocleidomastoid muscles of 6 COPD patients during sleep; the greatest loss of tone occurred during phasic REM and resulted in the most profound drop of oxygen saturation.

V/Q inequalities occur during sleep because FRC is reduced. FRC falls during sleep both because of the supine position assumed for sleeping and because of reduced chest wall movement resulting from REM sleep (Fletcher et al 1983, Hudgel et al 1983). V/Q inequalities worsen with reduced FRC if the end of the normal breath falls below the closing capacity. This can increase effective shunt, resulting in worsened hypoxemia during sleep. Indeed, venous admixture has been shown by Fletcher and colleagues (1983) to worsen during REM sleep in COPD patients. Another potential mechanism of V/Q mismatch during sleep is pooling of secretions; while sleeping, the patient coughs less frequently, secretions can accumulate, airways close, and V/Q mismatching results.

The end result for patients with COPD is hypoxemia during sleep, which is due primarily to hypoventilation (Becker et al 1999). Over 4 decades ago, Robin (1958) recognized that hypoxemia commonly occurs during sleep. Flick and Block (1977) were the first to monitor oxygen saturation (SaO_2) continuous with an ear oximeter. Numerous subsequent studies have clearly showed that hypoxemia is more severe for the COPD patients while asleep than awake and most severe of all during REM sleep (Douglas et al 1979, Littner et al 1980, Fleetham et al 1982). Further, the degree of nocturnal oxygen desaturation in patients with COPD can affect mortality (Kimura et al 1998). Unfortunately, however, Chaouat and colleagues (1997) concluded that the degree of nocturnal desaturation could not be predicted by any daytime variable except an elevated arterial carbon dioxide tension.

COPD Patients Sleep Poorly

In the Tucson Epidemiologic Study of Obstructive Airways Disease, 2,187 general population subjects (85% without and 15% with COPD) responded to questions about sleep symptoms (Klink and Quan 1994). Patients with chronic obstructive lung disease were more likely to endorse symptoms of initiating or maintaining sleep or excessive daytime drowsiness than were their age-matched counterparts. Forty-one percent of the COPD respondents had at least one symptom of disturbed sleep. Cormick and coworkers (1986) compared 50 COPD patients with 40 controls and showed that insomnia and daytime sleepiness were more common in the COPD patients. Investigators in the Cardiovascular Health Study have reported that individuals with self-reported emphysema experience more difficulty with frequent awakenings and early morning awakening than those without (Newman et al 1997). Polysomnography on a subgroup of the COPD patients demonstrated that sleep tended to be worse in those with the most oxygen desaturation. EEG studies of patients with COPD have demonstrated reduced sleep efficiency and total sleep time, delayed sleep onset, and frequent awakenings (Fleetham et al 1982, Littner et al 1980).

COPD, however, is not the only reason for poor-quality sleep in these patients. Aging, depression, poor sleep hygiene, and medications may also contribute. Ancoli-Israel and Roth (1999) showed that most people with insomnia do not seek help for the problem but self-medicate with alcohol or over-the-counter aids. Further, Meissner and colleagues (1998) documented that almost half of a group of mostly adult men admitted to a Veterans' Administration hospital had a significant sleep complaint when administered a questionnaire, but none of these patients' records included mention of any patient symptom related to sleep. It is important for the clinician caring for patients with any chronic illness to recognize that sleep disturbances are common in these groups, and comprehensive care means addressing sleep issues, as well.

Sleep Apnea, Aging, and COPD

Against the backdrop of deteriorating sleep in the aging COPD patient is the rising prevalence of SDB. In brief, although the prevalence of SDB increases with age, the peak prevalence of clinically significant obstructive sleep apnea (OSA) occurs in mid life, probably about age 55 (Bliwise 1993, Bixler et al 1998, Phillips et al 1994, Hoch et al 1990). One possible explanation for this is that individuals with significant sleep apnea may not survive to old age. Another explanation is that the peak prevalence of severe obesity (the single most important risk factor for OSA) is also in mid life. Further, congestive heart failure, cerebrovascular disease, and disturbed sleep become more prevalent with aging and can result in central sleep apneas. Many SDB events that are "counted" in population-based studies in older individuals are central apneas. Central apneas do not have the same prognostic significance or pathologic basis as do obstructive apneas (Bliwise, Bixler et al), although there is some overlap (Dowdell et al 1990).

There clearly is some "normal" increase in SDB with aging. Approximately one third of seniors meet the criterion of 5 or more SDB events per hour of sleep (Bliwise 1993, Hoch et al 1990, Phillips et al 1992). While it is not clear that older patients have less morbidity and mortality for a given level of SDB, it is clear that more of them meet this minimal standard (Ancoli-Israel and Coy 1994). Clearly, a different "cut point" needs to be used in the elderly.

In a study of mortality in OSA, He and colleagues (1988) showed that an apnea index greater than 20 predicted increased mortality in those aged under 50, but not those above 50. Although minimally defined OSA (AHI > 5) has not been shown to affect survival (Phillips et al 1992, Phillips et al 1994, Hoch et al 1990, Mant et al 1995, Berry et al 1987), mortality and morbidity do increase with increasing AHI in the elderly (Ancoli-Israel et al 1989, Bliwise et al 1998). For example, typical OSA pathology (sleepiness and cognitive dysfunction) appeared in our cohort of healthy seniors who met a cut point of AHI greater than 10 (Berry et al) and in a clinical geriatric population with a mean RDI of 37 (Levy et al 1996). In this context, it is important to note that African Americans over 65 have a two-fold risk of having an RDI greater than 30, with the corresponding clinical symptoms and increased risk of hypertension (Ancoli-Israeli et al 1995).

The "Overlap Syndrome"

Guilleminault and colleagues (1980) first described sleep studies of 26 COPD patients presenting to a sleep disorders center with daytime sleepiness. Of the 10 who had adequate sleep testing, 9 had significant OSA. Flenley (1985) later used the term "overlap syndrome" to refer to patients who have both COPD and OSA. In a study of 5,201 adults aged 65 and older, Enright and colleagues (1996) reported that observed apneas were associated with the presence of self-reported bronchitis in men.

The prevalence of mixed COPD and OSA is probably about 10% to 20% (Chaoaut et al 1995, Bradley et al 1986, Fischer and Raschke 1993). This is higher than what would be predicted simply by multiplying the rate of COPD (about 15%, according to Lebowitz [1989]) and OSA in an age-and-gender-matched cohort (31%, according to Young et al [1993]). Several factors probably account for the high prevalence of overlap syndrome. Both disorders predominantly affect older men. Further, cigarette smoking is a significant risk factor for both entities (Wetter et al 1994). It is also likely that COPD-induced derangements of respiratory control contribute to the development of OSA in some patients (Radwan et al 1995). Finally, sleep deprivation, so prevalent in patients with COPD, worsens obstructive sleep apnea (Persson and Svanborg 1996).

OSA, COPD, RLS, and the Aged

Restless legs syndrome (RLS) and periodic limb movements of sleep (PLMS) deserve mention here because of their association with OSA and their extremely high prevalence in the geriatric population (Ancoli-Israel et al 1985). RLS is a collection of symptoms and can be diagnosed by history. PLMS is defined by electromyographic criteria in the sleep laboratory. Although PLMS is present in about 80% of patients with RLS, it is neither necessary nor sufficient to make the diagnosis (Trenkwalder et al 1996). Recently, clinical criteria for the diagnosis of RLS have been developed. They are a desire to move the extremities, often associated with paresthesias/dysesthesias; motor restlessness; worsening of symptoms at rest with at least temporary relief by activity; and worsening of symptoms in the evening or night (Walters et al 1995). This disorder probably affects 10% to 15

% of the population and is strongly associated with increasing age, OSA, renal failure, anemia, many medications, cigarette smoking, and obesity (Lavigne and Montplaisir 1994). In a study of 222 consecutive adults (mean age 60 ± 14 years) admitted to a general medical ward in a Veterans Affairs tertiary care hospital, Meissner and colleagues (1998) documented that 21% had either restless legs, in a combination of leg jerks and leg kicking, or twitching during sleep, associated with a sleep complaint. In no instance was the presence of this symptom documented in the patients' medical records! This study points out that symptoms of RLS are common in sick patients. This diagnosis ought to be considered in geriatric or COPD patients presenting with sleeping difficulty.

Treatment Issues

Treatment of sleep problems in older, sick patients is difficult. Ancoli-Israel (1997) has succinctly outlined the basic principles. Nonpharmacologic approaches include a regular schedule (particularly rising time), no napping, exposure to bright outdoor sunlight, and avoidance of caffeine, alcohol, and stimulant medications near bedtime. A "nocturnal activities hour" (2-4 AM) is used in some institutions. Exercise has clearly been shown to be beneficial in promoting sleep in a group aged 50-76 (King et al 1997). Individuals who smoke cigarettes are more likely to report sleeping difficulties, and COPD patients who smoke should certainly be advised to quit in the strongest possible terms (Phillips and Danner 1995). Patients of all ages with COPD and/or SDB need to be advised not only to quit smoking but also to lose weight, if applicable. Many will sleep better in the lateral decubitus position or mostly upright in a recliner.

Although there is little evidence that melatonin can improve sleep of insomniacs younger than 65 years, it may be effective for disrupted sleep in the elderly. Melatonin levels decline with aging and are lower in elderly insomniacs than in age-matched controls. Goldberg (1997) demonstrated that both insomnia symptoms and wrist actigraphy show improvement in geriatric insomniacs following treatment with varying doses of melatonin. However, because it may affect vascular tone and the effective dose is probably much smaller than what is currently being sold in health food stores, melatonin should be used cautiously, if at all, in the elderly and always with the warning that it is not monitored by the FDA.

Treatment of RLS is by eliminating contributing factors, if possible. Dopaminergic agents, opiates, benzodiazepines, and anticonvulsants are among the many agents used successfully to treat this disorder. Its association with OSA is complex and treatment of OSA may relieve PLMS (Yamashiro and Kryger 1994).

Oxygen

Oxygen remains a mainstay of treatment for patients with COPD. Based on reports from the Medical Research Council (1981) and the Nocturnal Oxygen Therapy Trial Group (1980), 15 to 24 hours of oxygen per day (which almost always includes the sleep time) can reduce mortality, but 12 hours a day (nocturnal) oxygen is associated with twice the mortality of continuous oxygen. To investigate whether oxygen is beneficial to patients with isolated sleep hypoxemia, Fletcher and colleagues published two studies in 1992. Patients who had at lease one nocturnal episode of SaO_2 below 85% and no less than 5 minutes with SaO_2 below 90% were more likely to die than those who did not experience that degree of hypoxemia. In the second study, patients with hypoxemia at night (but not during the day) were randomized to receive nocturnal oxygen or sham treatment. Although pulmonary artery pressure fell in the oxygen-treated group, there was no difference in mortality at 3 years. According to Weitzenblum et al (1997), the currently available data do not justify the routine use of nocturnal oxygen in patients with nocturnal oxygen desaturation who do not qualify for oxygen by conventional criteria.

Pharmacologic Treatment

Several medications have been used to treat sleep-related hypoxemia in COPD. Series, Cormier and LaForge (1989) showed a modest improvement in sleep oxygenation using protriptyline in a small number of patients with COPD. As do most tricyclic antidepressants, protriptyline suppresses REM sleep, and this is its likely mechanism of improved SaO_2 in chronic lung patients. It can also cause urinary retention and is best avoided in older men for this reason. Almitrine has also been shown to improve nocturnal oxygen in COPD patients, but it has significant side effects (neuropathy) and its long-term effects are not well-studied (Gothe et al 1988). Medroxyprogesterone acetate gives an unpredictable response but is feminizing and carries a significant risk of deep venous thrombosis (Dolly and Block 1983). The studies by Man et al (1996) and by Molloy and McNicholas (1993) agree that theophylline improves oxygenation during sleep, but are at variance as to whether this xanthine causes improvement or deterioration in sleep. Beta agonists do not appear to improve either oxygenation or sleep (Man et al). Ipratropium bromide does appear to improve both oxygenation and sleep quality, according to a very recent study (Martin et al 1999).

Noninvasive Ventilatory Support

Hypoventilation is the major factor underlying sleep hypoxemia in COPD. Several investigators have applied noninvasive ventilation to patients with COPD. Although negative-pressure ventilation has been applied to these patients, it can worsen the obstructive sleep apnea component, is difficult to tolerate, and has been shown by Shapiro et al (1992) to not have a positive effect on outcomes such as quality of life or dyspnea.

Noninvasive positive pressure ventilation (NPPV), either continuous (CPAP) or bilevel (BiPAP), has become widely available, mostly because of its use in OSA patients. Bilevel pressure actually affords the ability to ventilate the patient, as pressure is lower on exhalation than on inhalation. Elliot and colleagues (1992) treated 8 patients for 6 months with bilevel pressure and reported improved sleep and improved oxygenation. In a crossover study comparing nocturnal oxygen with bilevel pressure plus oxygen in 14 patients, the combined treatment was superior to oxygen alone. Strumpf and colleagues (1991) undertook a 3-month crossover trail of 19 patients with COPD using BiPAP average pressures of 15/2. Only 7 patients were able to complete the trial, and no benefits were shown in day-time gas exchange, strength, exercise endurance, sleep quality and duration, or symptoms. Gay and coworkers (1996) had similarly disappointing results in 13 hypercarbic COPD patients; the dropout rate was high and no improvements were seen compared with the control group.

Two large retrospective trials (Leger et al 1994, Simonds and Elliott 1995) have evaluated the outcome of COPD patients treated with NPPV for up to 5 years. COPD patients are more likely to discontinue NPPV than are patients who are receiving this treatment for neuromuscular diseases, and their survival appears to be similar to that of patients who are treated with nocturnal oxygen alone.

Thus, the data on the use of NPPV in COPD are disappointing and somewhat conflicting. In a very recent review of the literature and Consensus Conference (Goldberg et al 1999), participants reached the following conclusions: NPPV appears better tolerated for patients with COPD than is negative pressure ventilation; patients with little or no CO_2 retention gain little benefit from NPPV; and patients with nocturnal oxygen desaturation are most likely to benefit from NPPV. They suggested the following indications for usage of NPPV in patients who have COPD: (1) symptoms such as fatigue, dyspnea, morning headache, (2) one of the following physiologic criteria: $PaCO_2$ greater than 55 mm Hg **or** $PaCO_2$ of 50-54 mm Hg with nocturnal oxygen saturation less than 88% for 5 minutes while on oxygen at 2 L/min **or** $PaCO_2$ of 50 to 54 mm Hg and hospitalization related to recurrent episodes of hypercapneic respiratory failure. The authors of these suggestions were careful to point out that "the evidence is conflicting and far from definitive" for the use of NPPV in COPD (ACCP consensus, Goldberg et al 1999, p. 529).

Because nasal CPAP is the mainstay of treatment for OSA, it has been applied to patients with the overlap syndrome by Sampol and colleagues (1996), who noted that higher levels of CPAP were needed to eliminate apneas when oxygen was concomitantly applied. To date, published reports of bilevel pressure treatment of the overlap syndrome are lacking.

Treatment of the Overlap Syndrome/OSA

Despite the confusion about what constitutes a "pathological" level of SDB in the elderly, clinically significant OSA certainly does exist in this age group. Given the debate about the clinical significance and putative benefits of treatment of OSA in general (Wright et al 1997), it is difficult to base diagnostic criteria or treatment decisions on a single level of SDB in this age group.

Certain conditions should raise concern about the possibility of OSA and need for treatment in older patients and in those with COPD. Although sleepiness per se is a worthless symptom in any age group, having an automobile accident or near-accident due to sleepiness should raise a red flag. Rehm and Ross (1995) have shown that drivers over 60 who are involved in road crashes are more likely to be at fault, more likely to have medical conditions, and less likely to be intoxicated than their younger counterparts. Thus, the older patient who is suspected of sleep apnea ought to be queried about car wrecks and near misses.

Hypertension is a common medical problem in the elderly and in patients with COPD, and whether to ascribe it to OSA and treat SDB on that basis is highly questionable. There is considerable debate about whether sleep apnea causes hypertension is any age group (Guilleminault and Robinson 1997), although the evidence points in the direction of a causal relationship. One criterion to apply to the older patient suspected of sleep apnea might be the presence of hypertension that is difficult to control.

The issue of sleep apnea and cognitive dysfunction is more clearcut. Severe SDB (AHI > 40) is associated with neuropsychological deficits, some of which may be reversible with treatment (Bliwise 1993, Redline et al 1997). However, milder levels of SDB (RDI 10-20) do not appear to cause cognitive dysfunction in the absence of sleepiness (Redline et al). Both Cheshire and colleagues (1992) and Kim and co-investigators (1997) found a correlation between AHI and neuropsychological test results. Psychomotor efficiency and visual vigilance appear to be most sensitive to SDB (Cheshire et al). Deterioration in cognitive performance correlates both with degree of hypoxemia and with degree of sleep fragmentation. For this reason, COPD and "overlap" patients may be particularly vulnerable. The association of SDB with dementia, then, depends on the degree of SDB. Kim et al (1997) estimate that an AHI of 15 is equivalent to the decrement of psychomotor efficiency associated with 5 additional years of age, or 50% of the decrement associated with hypnosedative use. Bliwise (1993) speculates that the dementia is of vascular origin because of the association between OSA and hypertension, arrythmias, and decreased cerebral perfusion. Although depression is frequently cited as a result of OSA (Reynolds et al 1985), Research Diagnostic Criteria-defined depression was no more common in elderly subjects with an AHI greater than 5 than in controls (although dementia was). These data suggest that evaluation and treatment of the older patient who has cognitive dysfunction and suspected sleep apnea would seem prudent. (Logistically, however, application of either polysomnography or nasal CPAP treatment is not easy in the demented patient).

Donohue and Lowethan (1997) define nocturia as urination at night associated with the interruption of sleep. It increases with age, affecting 80% of those 80 and older, and results from many causes. Nocturia is well associated with OSA and may improve with CPAP treatment.

Finally, there is the issue of whether or not to search for and to treat OSA in the elderly to prevent excess mortality. As outlined above, population-based studies of "healthy elderly" have tended not to find excess mortality associated with OSA that is found incidentally.

In sum, the findings of sleepiness leading to accidents, cognitive dysfunction, nocturia and perhaps hypertension in the elderly patient with mild levels (AHI < 20) of SDB might be reasonable indicators to attempt treatment. Patients who present with higher levels of SDB (AHI > 20 or 30) probably deserve a trial of treatment. It is important to remember, however, that it is the degree of oxygen desaturation and sleep disturbance, rather than the apneas and hypopneas themselves, that ultimately does the damage. Treatment decisions ought to take these variables into account.

Standard treatment of OSA is nasal CPAP, which has a compliance rate of approximately 50% in all age groups (Kribbs et al 1993). There is no evidence that older people or patients who have COPD are less compliant with CPAP than any other age group, but several factors, including milder levels of SDB (which is associated with poorer compliance), cognitive dysfunction, impaired sleep, RLS, the need to expectorate sputum, and nocturia might be expected to adversely affect compliance in this group. Nevertheless, CPAP is safe, reasonably inexpensive, and probably effective in reducing many of the sequelae of OSA.

Oral devices are indicated for mild sleep apnea, snoring, and sleep apnea in which no other form of treatment is available or tolerated. They are a particularly useful option for geriatric patients, and some of them can be made to fit over dentures (Schmidt-Nowara et al 1995).

Surgical treatment, most commonly uvulopalatopharyngoplasty (UPPP), is widely employed in patients who are CPAP intolerant. However, it has a success rate of approximately 50%, and an age greater than 50 is associated with poorer surgical outcome (Scher et al 1996). Further, the underlying medical condition of many COPD patients puts them at higher risk for general anesthesia. Noninvasive surgical procedures, eg, laser-assisted UPPP (LAUP), have not been well-evaluated yet, but appear to have a success rate comparable to that of scalpel UPPP (Walker et al 1995).

Hypnotics

Although conventional wisdom advises against the use of pharmacologic agents in the elderly and for those with disorders of respiratory control, the use of hypnotics among institutionalized patients is 34% (Morgan 1987). Among independently living individuals over the age of 65, benzodiazepine use is 12% for women and 9% for men (Whitney et al 1998). In a group of 222 veterans queried about sleep complaints at the time of admission to a general medical ward, 34% had a complaint of insomnia and one third of these were taking hypnotic medication (Meissner et al 1998). Thus, we actually have accumulated a fair amount of experience with hypnotic use in the sick and elderly without ever condoning it. Benzodiaze-pines probably do not increase the risk or severity of SDB in the elderly (Camacho and Morin 1995). Concerns about dependence and blunted respiratory drive have probably been significant factors in limiting benzodiazepine use in COPD patients. In truth, there are very little data documenting adverse complications in this situation, despite a wealth of somewhat covert clinical experience.

The Cardiovascular Health Study is an ongoing, prospective study of 5,201 adults, aged 65 and older, that was specifically designed to identify factors related to the onset and course of coronary heart disease and stroke. As part of the Cardiovascular Health Study, Newman and colleagues (1997) reported that benzodiazepine use was associated with daytime sleepiness in men and warned, "Not surprisingly...the use of benzodiazepines in our co-hort was associated highly with trouble falling asleep and, perhaps, with residual daytime sleepiness. Clinicians must consider these risk when pre-scribing benzodiazepines for older patients" (p. 6). The following year, the same investigators, this time led by Whitney (1998), reported more detail about sleepiness in this group of subjects. Using the Epworth Sleepiness Scale (Johns 1991), they more closely evaluated sleepiness in these sub-jects. In this study, they found no association between benzodiazepine use and sleepiness in men; in fact, the women who took benzodiazepines re-ported less daytime sleepiness. They then conservatively concluded, "[I]t is generally accepted that EDS is commonly observed in the elderly after hyp-notic use because of a "hangover" effect from the long half-life of many of these medications.... A clinical trial will be necessary to determine whether or not occasional use of hypnotics for insomnia results in more or less day-time sleepiness in the elderly" (p. 35).

A strange "disconnect" appears in our evaluation and treatment of sleeping difficulties in the sick and old. Walsh and Schweitzer recently (1999) reported 10-year trends in the treatment of insomnia. They noted 2 discouraging facts: (1) pharmacologic treatment of insomnia fell dramati-cally from 1987 to 1996, and (2) the use of antidepressants, notably tra-zadone, has grown substantially. The authors present evidence that the use of antidepressants in insomnia has grown because of concern about depend-ence rather than because of recognition and treatment of depression in those reporting insomnia. Trazadone is associated with significant side effects, including daytime somnolence, orthostatic dizziness/hypotension, and priapism (Nierenberg and Peck 1989, Thompson et al 1990). Further, trazadone appears to improve sleep in the non-depressed patient only in the short term and is less effective than zolpidem (Walsh et al 1998).

Development of newer hypnotics with inactive metabolites, short half-lives, and without respiratory depressive side effects renders the argument about benzodiazepine sleeping aids and their risk/benefit ratio in the elderly, terminal, and those with cardiopulmonary disease somewhat academic. A more germane issue is whether it is ethical to withhold such agents from terminal, sleepless individuals in whom efforts should be focused on comfort measures.

Sleeping difficulty, like pain, is probably inadequately evaluated and treated in terminal patients and in patients with COPD. New hypnotic agents have minimal side effects and excellent efficacy. We are missing opportunities to improve the quality of life in the end-stage COPD patient by failing to anticipate, ask about, evaluate, and treat sleeping problems.

References

Ancoli-Israel, S. 1997. Sleep problems in older adults: putting myths to bed. *Geriatrics.* 52:20-30.

Ancoli-Israel, S and T Coy. 1994. Are breathing disturbances in elderly equivalent to sleep apnea syndrome? *Sleep.* 17:77-83.

Ancoli-Israel, S, MR Klauber, DF Kripke et al. 1989. Sleep apnea in female nursing home patients: increased risk of mortality. *Chest.* 996:1054-1058.

Ancoli-Israel, S, MR Klauber, C Stepnowsky, E Estline, A Chinn, and R Fell. 1995. Sleep-disordered breathing in African-American elderly. *Am J Respir Crit Care Med.* 152:1946-1949.

Ancoli-Israel, S, DF Kripke, W Mason, and OJ Kaplan. 1985. Sleep apnea and periodic movements in an aging sample. *J Gerontology.* 40:419-425.

Ancoli-Israel, S and T Roth. 1999. Characteristics of insomnia in the United States: results of the 1991 National Sleep Foundation Survey. 1. *Sleep.* 22:S 347-353.

Becker, HF, AJ Piper, WE Flynn, SG McNamara, RR Grunstein, JH Peter, and CE Sullivan. 1999. Breathing during sleep in patients with nocturnal desaturation. *Am J Respir Crit Care Med.* 159:112-118.

Berry, DTR, BA Phillips, YR Cook, FA Schmitt, RL Gilmore, R Patel, TM Keener, and E Tyre. 1987. Sleep-disordered breathing in healthy aged persons: possible daytime sequelae. *J Gerontology.* 42:620-626.

Berry, DTR, BA Phillips, YR Cook, FA Schmitt, NA Honeycutt, AA Arita, and RS Allen. 1990. Geriatric sleep apnea syndrome: a preliminary description. *J Gerontology.* 45:169-174.

Bixler, EO, AN Vgontzas, TT Have, K Tyson, and A Kales. 1998. Effect of age on sleep apnea in men. *Am J Respir Crit Care Med.* 157:144-148.

Bliwise, DL. 1993. Sleep in normal aging and dementia. *Sleep.* 16:40-81.

Bliwise, DL, NG Bliwise, M Partinin, AM Pursley, and WC Dement. 1998. Sleep apnea and mortality in an aged cohort. *Am J Pub Hlth.* 78:544-547.

Bradley, TD, R Rutherford, F Lue et al. 1986. Role of diffuse airway obstruction in the hypercapnia of obstructive apnea. *Am Rev Respir Dis.* 134:920-924.

Brown, LK. 1998. Sleep-related disorders and chronic obstructive pulmonary disease. *Respir Care Clinics of N Amer.* 4:3(Sep):493-512.

Camacho, ME and CM Morin. 1995. The effect of temazepam on respiration in elderly insomniacs with mild sleep apnea. *Sleep.* 18:644-645.

Chaouat, A, E Weitzenblum, R Kessler, C Charpentier, M Ehrhard, P Levi-Valensi et al. 1997. Sleep-related desaturation and daytime pulmonary haemodynamics in COPD patients with mild hypoxemia. *Eur Respir J.* 10:1730-1735.

Chaouat, A, E Weitzenblum, J Kreiger, I Ifoundza, M Oswald, and R Kessler. 1995. Association of chronic obstructive pulmonary disease and sleep apnea syndrome. *Am J Respir Crit Care* Med. 151:82-86.

Cheshire, K, H Engleman, IA Dreary, C Shapiro, and NJ Douglas. 1992. Factors impairing daytime performance in patients with sleep apnea/hypopnea syndrome. *Arch Int Med.* 152:538-541.

Cooper, KR and BA Phillips. 1982. The effect of short-term sleep loss on respiration. *J Applied Physiology.* 53:855-858.

Cormick, W, LG Olson, MJ Hensley, and NA Saunders. 1986. Nocturnal hypoxemia and quality of sleep in patients with chronic obstructive lung disease. *Thorax.* 41:846-54.

Dolly, FR and AJ Block. 1983. Medroxyprogesterone acetate in COPD: Effect on breathing and oxygenation in sleeping and awake patients. *Chest.* 84:394-398.

Donohue, JL and DT Lowenthal. 1997. Nocturnal polyuria in the elderly person. *Am J Med Sci.* 314:232-238.

Douglas, NJ, PMA Calverly, RJE Leggett, HM Brash, DC Flenley, and V Brezinova. 1979. Transient hypoxemia during sleep in chronic bronchitis and emphysema. *Lancet.* I:1-4.

Douglas, NJ, DP White, CK Pickett, JV Weil, and CW Zwillich. 1982. Respiration during sleep in normal man. *Thorax.* 37:840-844.

Dowdell, WT, S Jahaveri, and W McGinnis. 1990. Cheyne-Stokes respiration presenting as sleep apnea syndrome. *Am Rev Respir Dis.* 141:871-879.

Elliott, MW, AK Simonds, MP Carroll et al. 1992. Domiciliary nocturnal nasal intermittent positive pressure ventilation in hypercapneic respiratory failure due to chronic obstructive lung disease: effects on sleep and quality of life. *Thorax.* 47:432-438.

Enright, PL, A Newman, P Wahl, T Manolio, E Haponik, and PJR Boyle. 1996. Prevalence and correlation of snoring and observed apneas in 5,201 older adults. *Sleep.* 19(7):531-538.

Fischer, J and F Raschke. 1993. Incidence of obstructive sleep apnea syndrome in combination with chronic obstructive respiratory tract disease. *Pneumologie.* 47 (suppl. 4):731-734.

Fleetham, J, P West, B Mezon, W Conway, T Roth, and MH Kryger. 1982. Sleep, arousals and oxygen desaturation in chronic obstructive pulmonary disease. *Am Rev Respir Dis.* 122:849-857.

Flenley, DC. 1985. Sleep in chronic obstructive lung disease. *Clin in Chest Med.* 6:651-661.

Fletcher, EC, CF Donner, B Midgren, J Zielinski, R Levi-Valensi, A Braghioroli, Z Rida, and CC Miller. 1992. Survival in COPD patients with a daytime $PaO_2 > 60$ mm Hg and without nocturnal oxyhemoglobin desaturation. *Chest.* 101:649-655.

Fletcher, EC, BA Gray, and DC Levin. 1983. Cardiopulmonary hemodynamics during sleep in subjects with chronic obstructive pulmonary disease: the effect of short and long term oxygen. *Chest.* 85:6-14.

Fletcher, EC, RA Luckett, S Goodnight-White, CC Miller, W Qian, and C Costarangos-Galarza. 1992. A double-blind trial of nocturnal supplemental oxygen for sleep desaturation in patients with chronic obstructive pulmonary disease and a daytime PaO$_2$ above 60 mm Hg. *Am Rev Respir Dis.* 145:1070-1076.

Flick, MR and AJ Block. 1977. Continuous in vivo monitoring of arterial oxygenation in chronic obstructive lung disease. *Ann Int Med.* 86:725-730.

Foley, DJ, AA Monjan, SL Brown, EM Simonsick, RB Wallace, and DG Blazer. 1995. Sleep complaints among elderly persons: an epidemiologic study of three communities. *Sleep.* 18:425-432.

Friedman, RC, DS Kornfield, and TJ Bigger. 1973. Psychological problems associated with sleep deprivation in interns. *J Med Ed.* 48:436-441.

Gay, P, RD Hubmayr, and RW Stroetz. 1996. Efficacy of nocturnal positive-pressure ventilation in stable, severe chronic obstructive pulmonary disease during a 3 month controlled trial. *Mayo Clinic Proceedings.* 71:533-542.

Goldberg, A, P Leger, N Hill, and G Criner. 1999. Clinical indications for noninvasive positive pressure ventilation in chronic respiratory failure due to restrictive lung disease, COPD, and nocturnal hypoventilation: a consensus conference report. *Chest.* 116(2):521-534.

Goldberg, JR, ed. 1997. *Is Melatonin a Treatment for Insomnia and Jet Lag? A White Paper of the National Sleep Foundation.* Washington, DC: NSF, 1997.

Gothe, B, NS Cherniack, RT Bachand, MB Szalkowski, and KA Bianco. 1988. Long-term effects of almitrine bimesylate on oxygenation during wakefulness and sleep in chronic obstructive pulmonary disease. *Am J Med.* 84:436-443.

Guilleminault, C, J Cummiskey, and J Motta. 1980. Chronic obstructive airflow disease and sleep studies. *Am Rev Respir Dis.* 122:397-405.

Guilleminault, C and A Robinson. 1997. Sleep-disordered breathing and hypertension: past lesions, future directions. *Sleep.* 20:806-811.

He, J, MH Kryger, FJ Zorick, W Conway, and T Roth. 1988. Mortality and apnea index in obstructive sleep apnea: experience in 385 male patients. *Chest.* 94:9-14.

Hoch, CC, CF Reynolds, TH Monk, DJ Buysse, AL Yeager, PR Houck, and DJ Kupfer. 1990. Comparison of sleep-disordered breathing among healthy elderly in the seventh, eighth, and ninth decades of life. *Sleep.* 13:502-511.

Hudgel, DW, RJ Martin, M Capeheart, B Johnson, and P Hill. 1983. Contribution of hypoventilation to sleep oxygen desaturation in chronic obstructive pulmonary disease. *J Applied Physiology.* 55:669-677.

Johns, MW. 1991. A new method for measuring daytime sleepiness. *Sleep.* 14:540-545.

Johnson, MW and JE Remmers. 1984. Accessory muscle activity during sleep in chronic obstructive pulmonary disease. *J Applied Physiology.* 57:1011-1017.

Kim, H, T Young, G Matthews, SM Weber, AR Woodard, and M Palta. 1997. Sleep-disordered breathing and neuropsychological deficits. *Am J Respir Crit Care Med.* 156:1813-1819.

Kimura, H, A Suda, T Sakuma, K Tatsume, Y Kawakami, and K Takayuki. 1998. Nocturnal oxyhemoglobin desaturation and prognosis in chronic obstructive pulmonary disease and late sequelae of pulmonary tuberculosis. *Int Med.* 37(4):354-359.

King, AC, RF Oman, GS Brassington, DL Bliwise, and WL Haskell. 1997. Moderate intensity exercise and self-rated quality of sleep in older adults. *JAMA.* 277:32-37.

Klink, M and SF Quan. 1994. The relation of sleep complaints to respiratory symptoms in a general population. *Chest.* 105:151-154.

Kribbs, NB, AI Pack, LR Kline, PL Smith, AR Schwartz, NM Schubert, S Redline, JN Henry, JE Getsy, and DF Dinges. 1993. Objective measurement of patterns of nasal CPAP use by patients with obstructive sleep apnea. *Am Rev Respir Dis.* 147:887-895.

Lavigne, GJ and J Montplaisir. 1994. Restless legs syndrome and sleep bruxism: prevalence and association among Canadians. *Sleep.* 17:739-743.

Lebowitz, MD. 1989. The trends in airway obstructive disease morbidity in the Tucson epidemiologic study. *Am Rev Respir Dis.* 140:S35-S41.

Leger, P, JM Bedicam, A Cornette, O Reybet-Degat, B Langevin, JM Polu, L Jeannin, and D Robert. 1994. Nasal intermittent positive pressure: long-term follow-up in patients with severe chronic respiratory insufficiency. *Chest.* 105:100-105.

Leighton, K and M Livingston. 1983. Fatigue in doctors. *Lancet.* 1:1280.

Levy, P, JL Pepin, D Malauzat, JP Emeriau, and JM Leger. 1996. Is sleep apnea syndrome in the elderly a specific entity? *Sleep.* 19:S29-S38.

Littner, MR, DJ McGinty, and DL Arand. 1980. Determinants of oxygen desaturation in the course of ventilation during sleep in chronic obstructive pulmonary disease. *Am Rev Respir Dis.* 122:849-857.

Man, CCW, KR Chapman, SH Ali, and AC Darke. 1996. Sleep quality and nocturnal respiratory function in once-daily theophylline (Uniphyl) and inhaled salbutamol in patients with COPD. *Chest.* 110:646-653.

Mant, A, M King, NA Saunders, CD Pond, E Goode, and H Hewitt. 1995. Four-year follow-up of mortality and sleep-related respiratory disturbance in nondemented seniors. *Sleep.* 18:433-438.

Marcus, CL and GM Loughlin. 1996. Effect of sleep deprivation on driving safety in housestaff. *Sleep.* 19:763-766.

Martin, RJ, BLB Bartelson, PL Smith, DW Hudgel, D Lewis, G Pohl, P Koker, and JF Souhrada. 1999. Effect of ipratropium bromide treatment on oxygen saturation and sleep quality in COPD. *Chest.* 115:1338-1345.

Martin, S, HM Engleman, IJ Dreary, and NJ Douglas. 1996. The effect of sleep fragmentation on daytime function. *Am J Respir Crit Care Med.* 1328-32.

Medical Research Council Working Party. 1981. Long-term domiciliary oxygen therapy in chronic hypoxic cor pulmonale complicating chronic bronchitis and emphysema. *Lancet.* 1:681-686.

Meissner, H, A Reimer, SM Santiago, M Stern, and MD Goldman. 1998. Failure of physician documentation of sleep complaints in hospitalized patients. *West J Med.* 169:146-149.

Meurice, JC, I Marc, and F Series. 1995. Influence on ventilatory and upper airway response to CO_2 in normal subjects and patients with COPD. *Am J Respir Crit Care Med.* 152:538-544.

Miles, L and WC Dement. 1980. Sleep and aging. *Sleep.* 3:119-220.

Molloy, E and WT McNicholas. 1993. Theophylline improves gas exchange during rest, exercise, and sleep in severe chronic obstructive pulmonary disease. *Am Rev Respir Dis.* 148:1030-1036

Morgan, K. 1987. *Sleep and Aging: A Research-Based Guide to Sleep in Later Life.* Baltimore, MD: The Johns Hopkins University Press.

Newman, AB, PL Enright, TA Manolio, EF Haponik, and PW Wahl. 1997. Sleep disturbance, psychosocial correlated, and cardiovascular disease in 5201 older adults: the cardiovascular health study. *J Am Geriatrics Soc.* 45:1-7.

Nierenberg, AA and PE Peck. 1989. Management of monoamine oxidase inhibitor-associated insomnia with trazadone. *J Clin Psychopharmacology.* 9:42-45.

Persson, HE and E Svanborg. 1996. Sleep deprivation worsens obstructive sleep apnea: comparison between diurnal and nocturnal polysomnography. *Chest.* 109:645-50.

Phillips, BA, DTR Berry, FA Schmitt, LG Harbison, and T Lipke-Molby. 1994. Sleep-disordered breathing in healthy aged persons: two and three year follow-up. *Sleep.* 17:411-5.

Phillips, BA, DTR Berry, FA Schmitt, LA Magan, DC Gerhardstein, and YR Cook. 1992. Sleep-disordered breathing in the healthy elderly: clinically significant? *Chest.* 101:345-349.

Phillips, BA, DTR Berry, FA Schmitt, R Patel, and YR Cook. 1989. Sleep quality and pulmonary function in the healthy elderly. *Chest.* 95:60-64.

Phillips, BA, KR Cooper, and TV Burke. 1987. The effect of sleep loss on breathing in patients with COPD. *Chest.* 9:29-32.

Phillips, BA and FJ Danner. 1995. Cigarette smoking and sleep disturbance. *Arch Int Med.* 155:734-737.

Radwan, L, Z Maszczyk, A Kziorowski, M Koziej, J Cieslicki, P Sliwinski, and J Zielinski. 1995. Control of breathing in obstructive sleep apnea and in patients with the overlap syndrome. *Eur Respir J.* 8:542-545.

Rediehs, MH, JS Reis, and NS Creason. 1990. Sleep in old age: focus on gender differences. *Sleep.* 13:410-424.

Redline, S, ME Strauss, N Adams, M Winters, T Roebuck, K Spry, D Rosenberg, and K Adams. 1997. "Neuropsychological function in mild sleep-disordered breathing." *Sleep.* 20:160-167.

Rehm, C and S Ross. 1995. Elderly drivers involved in road crashes: a profile. *Am Surgeon.* 61:435-437.

Reynolds, CF, DJ Kupfer, LS Taska, CC Hoch, DE Sewitch, K Restifo, DG Spiker, B Aimmer, R Marin, J Nelson, D Martin, and R Morycz R. 1985. Sleep apnea in Alzheimer's dementia: correlation with mental deterioration. *J Clin Psych.* 46:257-261.

Robin, ED. 1958. Some interrelationships between sleep and disease. *Arch Int Med.* 102:669-675.

Sampol, G, MT Sagales, A Roca , MD de la Calzada, JM Bofill, and F Morell. 1996. Nasal continuous positive airway pressure with supplemental oxygen in coexistent sleep apnea-hypopnea syndrome and severe chronic obstructive pulmonary disease. *Eur Respir J.* 9:111-116.

Scher, A, KB Schechtman, and JF Piccirillo. 1996. The efficacy of surgical modification of the upper airway in adults with obstructive sleep apnea syndrome. *Sleep.* 19:156-177.

Schmidt-Nowara, W, A Lowe, A Weigand, RC Cartwright, F Perez-Guerra, and S Menn. 1995. Oral appliances for the treatment of snoring and obstructive sleep apnea: a review. *Sleep*. 18:501-510.

Series, F, Y Cormier, and J LaForge. 1989. Changes in day and night time oxygenation with protriptyline in patients with obstructive pulmonary disease. *Thorax*. 44:275-279.

Series, F, N Roy, and I Marc. 1994. Effects of sleep deprivation and sleep fragmentation on upper airway collapsibility in normal subjects. *Am J Respir Crit Care Med*. 150:481-485.

Shapiro, SH, P Ernst, K Gray-Donald et al. 1992. Effect of negative pressure ventilation in severe chronic obstructive pulmonary disease. *Lancet*. 340:1425-1429.

Simonds, AK and MW Elliott. 1995. Outcome of domiciliary nasal intermittent positive pressure ventilation in restrictive and obstructive disorders. *Thorax*. 50:604-609.

Strumpf, DA, RP Millman, CC Carlisle et al. 1991. Nocturnal positive-pressure ventilation via nasal mask in patients with severe chronic obstructive pulmonary disease. *Am Rev Respir Dis*. 144:1234-1239.

Thompson, JW, MR Ware, and RK Blashfield. 1990. Psychotropic medication and priapism: a comprehensive review. *J Clin Psych*. 51:430-433.

Trenkwalder, C, AS Walters, and W Hening. 1996. Periodic limb movements and restless legs syndrome. *Neurology Clinics*. 14:629-650.

Walker, R, MM Grigg-Damberger, C Gopalsami, and MC Totten. 1995. Laser-assisted uvulopalatoplasty for snoring and obstructive sleep apnea: results in 170 patients. *Laryngoscope*. 105:938-943.

Walsh, JK, M Erman, CW Erwin, A Jamieson, M Mahowald, Q Regestein, M Scharf, P Tigel, G Vogel, and JC Ware. 1998. Subjective hypnotic efficacy of trazadone and zolpidem in DSM-III-R primary insomnia. *Human Psychopharmacology*. 13:191-198.

Walsh, JK and PK Schweitzer. 1999. Ten-year trends in the pharmacological treatment of insomnia. *Sleep*. 22:371-375.

Walters, AS and the International Restless Legs Study Group. 1995. Toward a better definition of restless legs syndrome. *Movement Disorders*. 10:634-642.

Weitzenblum, E, A Chaout, C Charpentier, M Ehrhart, R Kessler, P Schinkewitch, and J Kreiger. 1997. Sleep related hypoxaemia in chronic obstructive pulmonary disease: causes, consequences, and treatment. *Respiration*. 64:187-193.

Wetter, D, T Young, T Bidwell, MS Badr, and M Palta. 1994. Smoking as a risk factor for sleep-disordered breathing. *Arch Int Med*. 154:2219-2224.

White, JES, MJ Drinnan, AJ Smithson, CJ Griffiths, and CJ Gibson. 1995. Respiratory muscle activity during rapid eye movement (REM) sleep in patients with chronic obstructive pulmonary disease. *Thorax*. 50:376-382.

Whitney, CW, PL Enright, AB Newman, W Bonekat, D Foley, and SF Quan. 1998. Correlates of daytime sleepiness in 4578 elderly persons: the cardiovascular health study. *Sleep*. 21(1):27-52.1

Wilkinson, R. 1963. After affect of sleep deprivation. *J Experimental Psychology*. 66:439.

Wright, J, R Johns, I Watt, A Melville, and T Sheldon. 1997. The health effects of obstructive sleep apnoea and the effectiveness of treatment with continuous positive airway pressure: a systematic review of the research evidence. *Br Med J.* 314:851-60.

Yamashiro, Y and MH Kryger. 1994. Acute effect of nasal CPAP on periodic limb movements associated with breathing disorders during sleep. *Sleep.* 17:172-175.

Young, T, M Palta, J Dempsey, J Skatrud, S Weber, and S Badr. 1993. The occurrence of sleep-disordered breathing among middle-aged adults. *New Engl J Med.* 328:1230-1235.

19

Conversations With Patients About Palliative Care for Advanced COPD

Paul Fairman, MD, FACP, FCCP

Palliative care for patients with advanced chronic obstructive pulmonary disease (COPD) requires advance planning—the process of delineating those elements of medical care that a patient would and would not want as the disease progresses. At a minimum, advance planning will identify the person who can make decisions for the patient when the patient is unable to make them, but, more important, it will clarify for the proxy decision maker and for the health care providers the patient's wishes as they relate to future treatment. Palliative care for advanced COPD patients begins with advance planning that enlists the patient in structured conversations exploring his or her preferences for care and documenting them for all those who will aid the patient.

There are numerous logical reasons that would encourage physicians to aid patients with advanced COPD in creating an advance directive. COPD is a frequent cause of death and disability; however, the capacity to predict the course of the disease remains limited. Shortness of breath, worsening as the disease progresses, leads to severe disability, accompanied by social, emotional, and, frequently, financial hardships. Quality of life is diminished even for patients at a "stable" stage of the disease. Acute exacerbations of COPD increase the symptoms of the disease and the risk of dying. If intensified treatment is not sufficient during an acute exacerbation, a period of mechanical ventilation may prevent death. However, not every patient survives mechanical ventilation, and, occasionally, the course of ventilation is quite prolonged and recovery is accompanied by increased symptoms and a lower quality of life. In addition, the risk of dying in the year following mechanical ventilation is high. Finally, a small fraction of patients may not regain adequate respiratory function and may remain ventilator dependent indefinitely. Unfortunately, no clinical measurements predict which outcome awaits a patient who experiences an acute exacerbation. Additionally, patients who have had an acute exacerbation of COPD are frequently incapable of understanding, formulating, or communicating their preferences for therapeutic options, such as mechanical ventilation. Physicians and family members are not always able to accurately predict whether patients would decide for or against specific treatments. Professional organizations have published guidelines to encourage physicians to address end-of-life issues with patients. Legislative initiatives, such as the Patient Self-Determination Act of 1991, attempted to make all hospitalized patients aware of their right to create an "advance directive." Unfortunately, even among chronically ill nursing home patients, fewer than 30% have created such a directive.

These numerous reasons should encourage physicians to aid patients with the creation of advance directives. Why, then, does assistance with advance directives remain an infrequent element in bedside care? Ironically, answers to this question may include some the very reasons that advance directives could be so beneficial: the uncertainty of prognosis and a variance in the relative importance of quality and quantify of life to individual patients. Also, some physicians might worry that patient choices change too frequently to make the effort worthwhile (although many studies suggest that only 20% make many significant changes). Additionally, advance planning requires time that may not be easily found in busy practice situations (Emanuel 1995). Furthermore, both physicians and patients may be uncomfortable with addressing end-of-life issues (Tulsky et al 1995). Finally, the process touches on the relationship of the patient with his or her physician, the health care system, and family and loved ones and on the goals of each patient's life. Indeed, patients often have goals and concerns that are only indirectly related to their medical problems (Singer et al 1999). The care and support of loved ones, friends, coworkers, and religious congregations may be more meaningful and beneficial in the last phase of life than the efforts of health care providers. As a consequence, physicians may have difficulty initiating advance planning discussions and may perform the task poorly, if undertaken. (Sullivan et al 1996, Tulsky et al 1998).

This chapter suggests one approach to an initial conversation about advance planning between the physician and the patient to identify the patient's goals and wishes for managing his or her disease, its symptoms, and its complications. Good palliative care requires a regular program of discussions and documentation of revised patient preferences. The initial discussion, however, is the most difficult. The approach suggested here includes an agenda introduced by open-ended questions, and relies on active listening and empathetic responses. The goal of such a conversation is a patient-centered plan consistent with available medical options. An advance planning conversation is not about setting limits, although that often occurs. It is not an exercise of selecting between two choices: curative or palliative care. Rather, the conversation is an attempt to find what is good about both options as they relate to that particular patient. It is about managing the patient's illness in a way that improves his or her odds of achieving a satisfactory end-of-life experience. Advance planning is an exercise that requires effort from both the patient and physician. It does not guarantee a patient's final experiences, but it can initiate a process that could, and should, shape the end-of-life experience in ways that most closely meet the patient's wishes; without it, there is little chance of establishing the desired course to a specific outcome. The following approach for initiating and conducting a planning discussion has been developed from the personal experiences of the author with severely ill and dying patients and their family members and from the experiences of colleagues, as supported by a growing body of literature on communication skills and end-of-life care (Buckman 1992, Byock 1997, Lipkin et al 1995, Lo et al 1999, Suchman et al 1997). Although little research is currently available, better approaches to advance planning will be developed when detailed evaluations and studies similar to those that have improved the technical care available for many illnesses are applied to this phase of care.

The Goal of the Conversation

The goal of an advance planning conversation is to establish with the patient the kind of medical care that he or she wants and does not want. The plan that is developed should be put into writing. Legal documents, such as a durable power of attorney for health care, may be created, but the plan in its entirety need not be incorporated into a legal document. The essence of the conversation should be written down as a reminder of what was discussed and decided and as a guide to care. The plan may consist of just a few words or sentences that outline specific goals of or limitations to care. At a minimum, it should name the surrogate decisionmaker. The plan may include a statement about whether mechanical ventilation or cardiopulmonary resuscitation (CPR) should be administered, because both are frequent concerns of patients, families, and caregivers. It may designate who should be called during an emergency and where the patient will go for emergency care. Copies of the plan should be kept by the patient, surrogate decisionmaker, and physician(s); others, such as family members or caregivers, might be given copies as well. The contents of the plan should be openly discussed and reviewed at periodic intervals, in advance of any major intervention, and in conjunction with any change in the patient's condition or decisions.

Difficulties Specific to Patients With Advanced COPD

COPD is a chronic disease with variable but unremitting symptoms (dyspnea, cough, and sputum production) that are difficult to control. Acute episodes of worsening symptoms and gas exchange may result from infection, bronchospasm, cardiac decompensation, or other causes. Acute exacerbations not only increase symptoms but may threaten life if the disease is advanced. A 5-center study of over 4300 seriously ill patients was conducted, titled the Study to Understand Prognoses and Preferences for Outcomes and Risks of Treatments (SUPPORT). Connors et al (1996) reported on 1016 patients from the study who suffered acute exacerbations of COPD severe enough to result in hypercapnia (PCO_2 greater than 50 mm Hg). About one half of these hospitalized COPD patients reported significant and poorly controlled pain during the hospitalization. In-hospital mortality was 11% and 1-year mortality was 43%. Rehospitalization was common, 50% within the following 12 months. At 6 months, only 25% of the patients were alive and able to report a good or better quality of life; 50% of the survivors reported fair to poor quality of life because of troubling symptoms, impaired physiologic reserve, and dependence on others for one more necessities of daily living. This percentage was 4 to 5 times higher than expected in a general population. The study confirmed that advanced COPD patients are a population with poor health status and high mortality. Nevertheless, the prognoses for individuals within this group are extremely varied; some patients with COPD may live for years with hypercapnia or after an episode of acute respiratory failure requiring mechanical ventilation.

All of this makes patient and family counseling difficult. How is planning conceivable when long-term survival is possible even after a prolonged critical illness? Patients may ask, "What does the future hold? How long do I have? Will there be another crisis? How long could I live after a crisis?" They often have trouble grasping both the prolonged, declining course and the sudden life-threatening potential of seemingly minor events, such as influenza. Between crises, disease progression may be so slow that patients and family members may be able to ignore that the patients do, in fact, have a severe illness. This complicates efforts to enlist patients and families in advance planning. During a crisis, decision making is difficult for patients, family members, and medical teams. Crisis episodes usually focus on the technological efforts to save lives and are frequently and understandably devoid of advance planning. The slow decline of COPD patients and the intermittent crises that they face make advance planning and preparation for death difficult. The slow decline also means patients spend more time in a debilitated condition and often require assistance for a longer interval before death.

When to Begin the Conversation

Because advanced COPD is a disease characterized by significant symptoms and high mortality, advance planning ought to be a routine part of care. It is not. Because COPD is a disease with a long symptomatic decline, there should be numerous opportunities for discussing patient preferences for care when acute exacerbations strike. There are. However, human nature makes it easy to postpone these discussions when a patient is not acutely ill. Unfortunately, acutely ill patients are often incapable of competent decision making. Therefore, when should the conversation occur? It is never too soon. A discussion might be held shortly after the diagnosis of COPD. Also, any of the following criteria suggest an advanced stage of the disease and thus should serve as a reminder to initiate a discussion:

- Substantial symptoms (similar to New York Heart Association class III or IV), or "permanent impairment of activities of daily living" (Hansen-Flashen 1997).
- Severe impairment by spirometric measurement (the American Thoracic Society defines "severe COPD" as an FEV_1 less than 35% of the patient's predicted value).
- Poor oxygenation evidenced by the need for continuous oxygen supplementation.
- Hypercapnia with a PCO_2 greater than 48 mm Hg.
- Referral to rehabilitation (Heffner et al 1996).
- Prior to major therapeutic intervention (major surgery, chemotherapy, radiation).
- Expected mortality from any and all causes greater than 25% at 2 years.

Each of these criteria identifies patients with advanced COPD; these are patients for whom there is risk of death during an acute exacerbation. Notice that referral to hospice is not one of the criteria. Advance planning discussions should precede such a referral, and published criteria for referral of COPD patients to hospice are not effective in identifying a population with a survival prognosis of less than 6 months (Fox et al 1999).

If physicians are uneasy with initiating conversations about end-of-life issues and advance planning, they should take comfort in knowing that available data, although limited, show that patients are overwhelmingly interested in such discussions. Heffner et al (1996) interviewed patients referred to a pulmonary rehabilitation program. Such patients generally have severe chronic lung disease but are not at the "end stage"; indeed, the referral suggests that both physicians and patients are actively seeking ways to improve the patients' functional status and quality of life. Such patients have not "given up." These patients were uniformly interested and willing to discuss end-of-life issues and planning. Therefore, physicians' concerns about introducing the issues surrounding dying should be reduced. Patients generally seem willing to participate in such discussions.

Getting Started

The language used is particularly important when discussing difficult topics such as setting goals and plans. Physicians of COPD patients should be aware of the unintended meanings that some common phrases may imply, such as "Do you want me to do everything possible?" or "What do you think about aggressive therapy?" Patients may interpret such statements to mean that their doctors think they should receive less than routine care or perhaps even that the patients will be abandoned. To assist discussions, the following approach includes suggested sentences and phrases as good beginnings to various portions of the advance planning conversation. Most are in the form of questions and are open-ended, requiring more than a few words in response from the patients. The suggested wording calls on patients to name their areas of concern. Because the questions and responses may touch on very personal values, hopes, or fears, emotions may run high during such a conversation. Whenever strong emotions surface, physicians should be prepared to wait quietly as the wave of emotion (sadness, anxiety, anger, blame, fear, denial, guilt, or shame) crests and falls. A statement that acknowledges the emotion or asks for a description of what the patient is feeling sends a strong message of support. Physicians should allow all of the emotional wave to be spent before moving further in the discussion.

Getting started may be the most awkward step in the process of advance planning. How can the topic be introduced in a way that does not immediately generate fear and anxiety in patients? While the question is appropriate, the concern may be exaggerated. As noted earlier, patients usually are interested in the topic and if given the opportunity with an open-ended question such as "Are there concerns we have not addressed yet?" or "Do you have any other questions?" may bring up the subject themselves. If not, a statement such as "It's good to work for and hope for the best, but it's wise to prepare for the worst. Let's consider what could happen if you become severely ill" may initiate a discussion. Such a statement is an appropriate part of the plans for the care of a patient and logically follows other parts of the plan of care, such as medication and/or oxygen prescription, infection prophylaxis, and rehabilitation. Perhaps the part of advance planning easiest to introduce is the idea of a surrogate decisionmaker (Gallagher et al 1999). A physician might ask, "Have you thought about who I can turn to for help if you are so ill that you cannot make decisions?" While the spouse is usually named, other options might be suggested if that individual is frail or otherwise incapable of making decisions. Whoever is named should be present for any additional advance planning. If that person is not present, and perhaps even if they are, the patient should be given some time to think about the issue. The physician might say, "I would like to make sure that you have time to think about this topic, that we have sufficient time to discuss it, and that your wife (or husband, child, friend, etc.) can be present for the meeting. So let's schedule a time for our discussion." In notifying the patient that there are additional important decisions to be made and providing the patient with an opportunity to gather his or her thoughts, the discussion may be facilitated.

Whether the advance planning discussion follows immediately or is scheduled for a later time, a good environment will help the conversation. Ample time in a private, quiet space without distractions is important. The patient's designated surrogate decisionmaker should be present. Everyone should be seated and comfortable and close enough for a reassuring touch if needed. The physician should be prepared to provide information about COPD, its treatments, and their benefits, burdens, and probable outcomes in simple, clear language. The physician should have several goals in mind, including naming a surrogate decisionmaker and clarifying the patient's thoughts about mechanical ventilation and CPR, but other concerns may arise. If not all areas can be addressed in the allotted time, a continuation of the conversation can be scheduled at a later date.

Determining the Patient's Understanding

Having planned and scheduled the visit and having created a good environment, beginning the conversation is often surprisingly easy. An opening question from the physician such as "What have you been thinking about this meeting?" may initiate a series of thoughts from the patient. At this point it is especially important for the physician to postpone providing in-depth answers to questions and volunteering large amounts of information. The goal for now is to hear the patient's view, to identify his or her concerns, and to elicit as much as the patient is prepared to divulge. Probing further, the physician should check for the patient's understanding of COPD and its likely outcome, perhaps through questions such as "What do you know about what people go through with this disease?" The answers to such open-ended questions and any brief questions to clarify can illustrate how much the patient already knows about COPD and its course. Whether the patient has the basic facts about COPD or needs additional instruction, such questions identify the starting point for the next step in the process.

In a similar fashion, the patient's knowledge of treatment options should be probed with an open-ended question such as "What treatment options are you aware of that we have if your disease should become worse?" Responses to the patient's statements should build on, adjust, or correct his or her understanding of COPD, its course, and its outcome. No effort should be made to soften or "sugar coat" the information; neither should it be made "darker" than the specifics of the disease. While the wide variability of disease progression and outcomes of acute exacerbations may seem dauntingly impossible to convey, it should be feasible to provide best and worst case scenarios with statements of the benefits and burdens associated with each. The patient will also want some idea of how likely each of the outcomes might be. Dales et al (1999) created a brief description of intubation and mechanical ventilation as a tool for helping patients make an informed decision about this particular issue. The language is simple and the statistics are kept to a minimum. Some patients will want more information before a decision, but Dales' description is an example of brief, clear material that could be provided as a foundation for understanding and decision making.

Identifying the Patient's Point of View

Once it is clear that a patient has sufficient knowledge about COPD and its treatments and probable outcomes, the next step should be to identify the patient's perspective. The physician may ask, "What is your understanding of where things stand now with your illness? As you think about the illness, what is the best and the worst that might happen? What are your goals, expectations, hopes, or fears for the future? What part of this illness has been most difficult for you?" It may take the patient a moment or two to organize his or her thoughts and begin to respond to questions like these. Active listening techniques, such as patience and silence, will help the patient to answer. A simple nod, yes, or um hmmm or "Is there anything else?" will elicit a more complete response, perhaps with other concerns or thoughts. It is good to hear all the patient's thoughts before substantively replying to any one of them. Jotting down the concerns or responses will facilitate discussing them all at a later point. Specific interventions, such as mechanical ventilation or CPR, need not be addressed at this point. The patient's surrogate decisionmaker should also be questioned about his or her concerns: "What has been on your mind as you think about this disease progressing?" The surrogate should also be given the opportunity to answer fully, with the same kind of active listening responses.

Once the patient's point of view has been elicited and the surrogate's concerns identified, each subject can be addressed individually. Whenever possible, it is valuable to begin each topic with the patient's own words: "You said you were afraid of suffocating; let's talk some more about that and what we can do about it." Using a few of the patient's words in your response gives the patient assurance that you were listening and accurately heard his or her concerns. It can also provide the common ground on which further understanding of the disease can be built.

Setting Goals

A patient's decisions about specific treatment options (mechanical ventilation, hospice care, etc.) may require enumerating the relative benefits and burdens of each treatment but also will require that the patient's goals and values be known. If a patient is having trouble articulating his or her goals, it may be beneficial to suggest possibilities. Singer et al (1999) interviewed patients whose projected risk of dying was high and asked what goals were important to them. These open-ended interviews were evaluated and the patients' comments categorized into several themes. The 5 most frequently mentioned goals were:

1. To receive adequate pain and symptom management.
2. To avoid inappropriate prolongation of dying.
3. To achieve a sense of control.
4. To relieve burdens on loved ones.
5. To strengthen relationships with loved ones.

This list may help a patient articulate personal goals and create a plan that supports them. It might be introduced by saying, "I want to ensure that you receive the kind of treatment that meets your goals. Do any of these statements describe one or more of your goals?" The list also has additional value in that it may reflect the features of the last stages of illness and dying that characterize in some way a "good death." Journalist Marilyn Webb (1998) observed patients as death neared and interviewed them and their families and friends. From her observations, she was able to identify characteristics frequently found in satisfying and meaningful end-of-life experiences. The characteristics include many of the concerns of patients near death, suggesting some core features that are truly meaningful to patients:

1. Sophisticated symptom control
2. Limits on excessive treatment
3. Preservation of the patient's decisionmaking power
4. Open, ongoing communication
5. Focus on preserving the patient's quality of life

Some of the patient's goals may be contradictory (prolongation of life and avoidance of mechanical ventilation, for example). Identifying these contradictions for a patient should lead to a clarification about which goal is primary or when one should take precedence over another. In addition, depending on the course of the disease or the response of the patient to the treatment, goals or the relative weight given to a particular goal may change. This may follow an event in the illness, such as failure of dyspnea to be improved by intensified bronchodilators with subsequent loss of mobility, or events in the family or patient's circle of support, such as a granddaughter's marriage or a spouse's illness. Whenever changes in goals may be expected to occur, goals and plans should be clarified, with questions such as "What are you hoping for now? What is most important now in your life? Is there anything that you are afraid of now?"

At the very least, hearing a patient's list of hopes, fears, goals, and concerns provides a starting place for further interventions. This list, like a medical problem list, can focus attention on the steps needed to address specific concerns. If some of the patient's goals are unrealistic, a more manageable goal may be identified. Goals can be checked, updated, and amended as the patient's situation changes.

The Mechanical Ventilation Question

If every concern cannot be addressed in a single planning session with a patient with advanced COPD, there is no issue, with the exception of naming a proxy decisionmaker, that is as important as establishing a patient's wishes concerning the use of mechanical ventilation. For COPD patients, episodes of acute respiratory failure are often defined by decisions about this major intervention. Life-saving in many instances, mechanical ventilation is also the epitome of many patients' worst fears. Sullivan et al (1996) documented the fact that the issue is not without emotional impact for physicians either, some of whom may have so strong an opinion that they frame their discussions with patients to facilitate a particular decision. To avoid such bias and to aid patients in their deliberations and decision making, Dales and colleagues (1999) devised a document that describes the rationale, benefits, and burdens associated with mechanical ventilation. Experience using the document is small, but preliminary results suggest that patients were able to make confident, satisfying decisions that were consistent over time. It may prove to be a valuable aid to decision making.

While mechanical ventilation decisions are important, they are, however, only one element in a plan of care that should encompass many facets. Hansen-Flashen (1997) suggests placing the mechanical ventilation question in a broader framework, consisting of 4 options for care:

- Home care only.
- Hospitalization, if necessary for comfort, but with no mechanical ventilation or major organ support provided.
- Full life support (including ventilation), to be continued only so long as there is a chance of recovery to independence.
- Indefinite support, even to the point of long-term ventilation, but only if cortical function is good.

The options are sufficiently different enough to give patients distinct choices but not so specific that a discussion about the choices would be excessively long or burdensome. This framework may help physicians and patients chart an appropriate course through the multiple decisions that accompany severe illness.

The CPR Question

Prognoses for many illnesses, even for those patients very near death, are ambiguous. Rather than counsel patients about a progressive downward trajectory, a better goal might be to ensure that patients understand the limits of medical intervention in prolonging life and what can be done to help prevent suffering or uncomfortable symptoms. CPR represents an excellent example of the limits of medical intervention. Contrary to popular belief and media depictions, CPR is a technique that is acutely successful (return of spontaneous heartbeat) for hospitalized patients in about 30% of attempts. Its "long-term" success (survival to discharge from the hospital) is about one third of the immediate success rate. Furthermore, the burdens of "success" are substantial: ICU care, mechanical ventilatory support, and almost certain loss of some neurologic function. In-hospital CPR fails (the patient dies) about 85% of the time, whereas most of the public believe that the success rate is 85%. Consent for CPR cannot be informed unless patients are aware of the outcomes and burdens of treatment. The topic might be introduced by saying, "Many patients with advanced COPD decline CPR. I wonder if you might be one of them. Let me tell you what it is, what it offers, and what its burdens are."

The Next Steps

Whatever decisions are made in an advance planning conversation, the discussion should conclude with a physician summary (a document that can be shared by both the physician and patient) and with a plan for any agreed on immediate steps and a scheduled follow-up appointment.

A major deficiency in advance planning is the potential lack of timeliness. Physicians and patients tend to view the decisions made at one point in time and under one set of conditions as permanent and immutable. Over the course of a chronic illness such as COPD, changing conditions may alter a patient's point of view. Some goals may have been reached; new ones may have appeared. The relative importance of major features in the advance directive may shift. New concerns may arise. Therefore, the plan must be reviewed with the patient and updated periodically and with any major event in the patient's course of treatment. Each update should be shared with the surrogate decisionmaker and other concerned family members or professionals.

Advance planning cannot address every medical possibility. Efforts to make the process achieve this end will routinely be frustrated. Physicians, patients, or families who expect no additional discussions or review of plans at the time of a medical crisis will be disappointed. However, advance planning focuses the goals of care and provides the framework for the specific decisions that are unique to an illness.

Summary

Introducing an advance planning discussion to a patient with advanced COPD may be difficult, but the approach outlined in this chapter has been well received by many patients:

- Create a good environment for the discussion.
- Use open-ended questions to determine what the patient knows about the disease and its treatment.
- Identify a surrogate decisionmaker.
- Elicit the patient's point of view and goals.
- Create a plan based on the patient's goals, including his or her decision about mechanical ventilation and CPR.
- Review the plan and the patient's goals at regular intervals and with changes in the disease or the patient's condition.

References

Buckman, R. 1992. *How to Break Bad News: A Guide for Health Care Professionals.* Baltimore, MD: Johns Hopkins University Press.

Byock, I. 1997. *Dying Well: The Prospect for Growth at the End of Life.* New York, NY: Riverhead Books.

Connors, AF, NV Dawson, C Thomas et al. 1996. Outcomes following acute exacerbation of severe chronic obstructive lung disease. *Am J Respir Crit Care Med.* 154:959-967.

Dales, RE, A O'Conner, P Hebert et al. 1999. Intubation and mechanical ventilation for COPD: development of an instrument to elicit patient preferences. *Chest.* 116:792-800.

Emanuel, L. 1995. Structured advance planning: is it finally time for physician action and reimbursement? *JAMA.* 274:510.

Fox, E, K Landrum-McNiff, Z Zhong et al. 1999. Evaluation of prognostic criteria for determining hospice eligibility in patients with advanced lung, heart, or liver disease. *JAMA.* 282:1638-1645.

Gallagher, TH, SZ Pantilat, B Lo, and MA Papadakis. 1999. Teaching medical students to discuss advance directives: a standardized patient curriculum. *Teaching & Learning in Med.* 11(3):142-147.

Hansen-Flashen, J. 1997. Palliation and terminal care. *Clin Chest Med.* 18:645-655.

Heffner, J, B Fahy, L Hilling et al. 1996. Attitudes regarding advance directives among patients in pulmonary rehabilitation. *Am J Respir Crit Care Med.* 115:639.

Lipkin, M, SM Putnam, and A Lazare, eds. 1995. *The Medical Interview.* New York, NY: Springer Verlag.

Lo, B, T Quill, and J Tulsky. 1999. Discussing palliative care with patients. *Ann Int Med.* 130:744-749.

Singer, PA, DK Martin, and M Kelner. 1999. Quality end-of-life care: patient perspectives. *JAMA.* 281:163-168.

Suchman, AL, K Markakis, HB Beckman, and R Frankel. 1997. A model of empathic communication in the medical interview. *JAMA.* 277:678-682.

Sullivan, KE, PC Hebert, J Logan et al. 1996. What do physicians tell patients with end-stage COPD about intubation and mechanical ventilation? *Chest.* 109:258-264.

Tulsky, JA, MA Chesney, and B Lo. 1995. How do medical residents discuss resuscitation with patients? *J Gen Int Med.* 10:436-442.

Tulsky, JA, GS Fischer, MR Rose, and RM Arnold. 1998. Opening the black box: how do physicians communicate about advance directives? *Ann Int Med.* 129:441-449.

Webb, M. 1996. *The Good Death.* New York, NY: Bantam Books.

20

End-of-Life Decisions in A1AD: Results of a Survey

Sandra K. Brandley, CRT, and Mary Pat Raimondi, MA

Health care providers struggle with providing meaningful care to patients in the end stages of life. Current hospice programs are tailored to provide care to meet the needs of patients with cancer, rather than more unpredictable diseases like lung, liver, and heart disease. This chapter will discuss the characteristics of this genetic disorder and the comments and end-of-life wishes of the unique population of those affected by alpha 1-antitrypsin deficiency.

What Is Alpha 1-Antitrypsin Deficiency?

First described in 1963 by Laurel and Ericksson, alpha 1-antitrypsin deficiency (A1AD) is a genetic condition estimated to affect 60,000 to 100,000 people in the United States. Evidence for this estimate is derived from several population-based screening studies and an additional study of 965 individuals with emphysema, in which 2% to 3% were diagnosed with A1AD (Stoller 1997). Despite its relatively frequent occurrence, the disorder is often underrecognized and underdiagnosed.

In a survey mailed to the readership of the *Alpha-1 News* (the national newsletter of the Alpha 1 Association), Stoller et al (1994) reported that 43.7% of the respondents indicated having seen three or more physicians before the diagnosis of A1AD was made. The respondents, whose mean age was 48.8 years, reported a mean age of onset of symptoms of 35 years and an average delay of 7 years between the time symptoms appeared and a definitive diagnosis was made.

The Alpha 1 Association, a grassroots patient advocacy organization with an international membership, estimates that fewer than 6000 of the projected 100,000 affected individuals in the United States are currently diagnosed. Clearly there is a wide discrepancy between prevalence and diagnosis; several possibilities for this discrepancy exist. A1AD's clinical presentation may be one of three distinctly different diseases: emphysema, cirrhosis of the liver, or panniculitis. Emphysema is by far the most common presentation of A1AD in adults. A1AD is also the most common genetic cause of liver disease and liver transplantation in infants and children, usually manifested as cirrhosis of the liver (Perlmutter 1995). (Cirrhosis of the liver in adults is much less common than in infants or children.) Panniculitis, a skin disorder, is the rarest manifestation.

According to Buist (1990), clinical histories for 120 patients with a diagnosis of A1AD and of pulmonary symptoms revealed 98% reporting dyspnea, 34% reporting chronic bronchitis, and 20% reporting reactive airways. With this evidence, an initial diagnosis of asthma, chronic bronchitis, or year-round allergies is understandable. Unfortunately, physicians often may not entertain a diagnosis of A1AD because of a misunderstanding of the frequency of the disorder. Perhaps that is the reason, as commonly reported by members of the Alpha 1 Association, for the unremitting and unresponsive nature of the symptoms to usual medical regimens.

Unlike the later onset of smoking-acquired emphysema, lung damage from A1AD, primarily evident in the lower lobes of the lungs, tends to appear in the third to fourth decades of life and it is a frequent cause of early retirement due to medical disability (Stoller 1994). This disease strikes young adults in their prime child-rearing and earning years. It is responsible for panacinar emphysema that frequently renders the affected individual eligible for a lung transplant. Trulock (1996) reports 13% of all lung transplants are performed because of A1AD.

Despite a potentially fatal disease occurring at a time so classically devoted to family and career, a significant number of respondents in the Alpha 1 News readership survey reported positive outcomes (Stoller 1994). Twenty-two percent reported an improvement in their marriage and 46.4% reported making new friends. However, positive attitudes notwithstanding, 75.3% of the respondents reported having had at least one adverse psychosocial effect, 44.4% having retired early, and 19.1% having changed to a less physically demanding job.

The Registry of Patients with Severe Deficiency of Alpha 1-Antitrypsin (sponsored by the National Heart, Lung and Blood Institute, National Institutes of Health) concluded a 7-year study in April 1996 (Alpha 1-Antitrypsin Deficiency Registry Study Group 1998). Out of 1026 patients enrolled, 147 deaths occurred during the study. Cause of death information was gathered on 118 individuals: emphysema in 85 cases (72%) and cirrhosis in 12 others (10%). Less frequent causes for death were malignancy (3), diverticulitis (2), sepsis/infection (2), and trauma/accident (2). The remaining 12 deaths were each attributed to a different cause.

End-of-Life Decisions Survey

Method of Data Collection

The end-of-life decisions survey was administered through "The International Alpha 1 Mailing List," an Internet list for people with A1AD. Many people who communicate via this list are homebound because of their disease; others do not have access to face-to-face support groups for the disorder or find the convenience of an Internet mailing list appealing. The mailing list is a virtual support group of over 500 members. Thirty-two completed surveys were received, for a 6% response rate. The demographics of the on-line respondents showed a nearly even distribution between men (46.9%) and women (53.1%). There was a uniform age spread for the most part. We received a 6.3% return from respondents aged 25-34 years, 21.9% from those aged 35-44 years, 34.4% from those aged 45-54 years, and an equal percentage (34.4%) from those aged 55-65 years. Twenty-five percent of the respondents had three or more members in their family. Many respondents had attained a higher level of education, with 59.4% of them having completed some college work or having received college degrees.

Survey Results

- People who had known about their A1AD longer were expected to be more likely to respond to a survey on end-of-life decisions. Surprisingly, however, there was an even distribution in the "length of diagnosis" category: 28.1% had been diagnosed for less than 3 years; 21.9% diagnosed for 3-5 years; 21.9% diagnosed for 5-10 years; and 28.1% diagnosed for over 10 years.
- The majority of respondents (81.2%) are seeing a pulmonologist as their primary care physician, or as a consultant with their internist or family practitioner. While 59.4% felt that their physicians were able to explain aspects of the disease with them, 53.1% of those surveyed reported that their physicians were not very knowledgeable about A1AD. Comments from respondents reflected this:

  "I was diagnosed for 5 years prior to being assigned this internist as my primary care, so I feel like I am leading her learning experience, rather than her me."

  "He is my fourth MD. How does one explain it?"

  "My family practice doctor never heard of Alpha. I gave [him] information. My pulmonary specialist gave [me] limited information, but I was on my own to get detailed information from the Internet."

  "I educated myself about this condition, then searched for an MD who knew at least as much about the condition as I had been able to get from medical libraries, the people on the Internet, and MDs connected to the various Alpha groups."

- Nearly all (96.9%) of the respondents reported experience with someone close to them dying, but only 25.1% felt that death was peaceful, well-prepared, or spiritual; 28.1% described the death negatively as lingering, prolonged, or sudden. An additional 6.3% felt that excessive medical treatment had been given their loved one. One respondent replied: "I have no fear of death but I am terrified of dying while under the care of the medical community. The loss of personal dignity to be witnessed by loved ones, the prolonged suffering in the name of 'good medicine,' the interaction with a distant professional, the financial burden of useless procedures are all deeply offensive to me. If I had the courage, I would walk in front of a Mack truck today to avoid this final reality of tomorrow." Conversely, 68.8% of the respondents felt that very caring or somewhat caring treatment had been offered their loved one.

- Of those surveyed, half responded to having living wills for themselves and 8 in 10 of those have discussed the documents with their families, but only 4 in 10 have discussed their living wills with their physicians. Yet, 62.5% felt that end-of-life decisions should be made based on discussions between family, patient, and physician. An additional 15.6% would add the patient's spiritual adviser to the discussion. Only 6.3% felt that only the patient should be consulted for end-of-life decisions. In answer to a separate question, 21.9% of respondents either agreed strongly or somewhat agreed that the physician should be the only one in charge of end-of-life decisions. Additionally, 78.1% of the group felt that their relationship with their physician was good or very good.

- Nearly 60% expressed a fear of dying, but also felt that they would prefer dying at home (62.5%). Comments included "I fear suffocating and I don't want to be on a respirator to live." Only 18.8% preferred a hospice setting. Comments written about fear of death were often cloaked in dark humor, such as the following: "I also have a fear of being buried. I prefer to become a cadaver so I can be cut to pieces by medical students, or used as a human crash test dummy. Then I can be fried to the point of extra, extra crispy, crushed into a fine dust, and tossed to the wind."

- Respondents were asked which issues would be important to them when facing death, and to rank them in order of importance. Preferences, from most important to least important, were: (1) relationships with loved ones, (2) management of breathlessness, (3) pain management, (4) having wishes respected, (5) having input into care, and (6) knowing that financial issues are settled. Expounding on the top-ranked issue, one patient said, "What is so hard to deal with ... is [wondering] what will happen to my family when I'm not here for them. My biggest concerns are for my children's future. I will fight this disease every step of the way and try to clear the path for others behind me to make it easier. I want to be here on this earth to see my grandchildren, and [I] have to face the possibility that I may not be here for that."

These findings are very similar to those of a study of three other patient groups: dialysis patients, HIV/AIDS patients, and long-term care patients (Singer 1999). Authors of that study concluded that such preferences could serve as focal points for improvement of the care of individuals at the end of life, a conclusion reinforced by the findings of the End-of-Life Decisions Survey.

- Respondents *unanimously* stated that they would like all possible information on their disease and situation, and thereby limit surprises. To meet this goal, the knowledge of physicians and other medical professionals involved in the care of A1AD must increase. A more comprehensive understanding of this disorder would also enable earlier diagnosis, which may allow alterations in health habits and lifestyle choices to prolong good health.

Conclusion

Thirty years since the identification of this common genetic disorder, many patients believe their physicians are not very knowledgeable about the disease. Clearly, ways must be found to provide professionals with the information they need to engender confidence in the care they offer. Several patient education gaps have been identified: patients are not discussing their end-of-life wishes with their physicians, yet expect them to play a major role in the execution of those wishes; and many patients wish to die in familiar surroundings, but are not informed on the option of hospice.

Those with A1AD are eager partners in their health care and in end-of-life decisions. "[F]or the patient to optimally benefit and for clinicians to feel confident in the care they provide, it is essential that the approach to a patient who is suffering in their dying be preceded by thoughtful preparation" (Byock 1996). We must be up to the task.

References

The Alpha 1-Antitrypsin Deficiency Registry Study Group. 1998. Survival and FEV$_1$ decline in individuals with severe deficiency of alpha 1-antitrypsin. *Am J Respir Crit Care Med*. 158:49-59.

Buist, AS. 1990. Alpha 1-antitrypsin deficiency—diagnosis, treatment, and control: identification of patients. *Lung*. Suppl:543-551.

Byock, IR. 1996. The nature of suffering and the nature of opportunity at the end of life. *Clinics in Geriatric Med*. (May) 12, 2:237-252.

Laurell, CB and S Eriksson. 1963. The electrophoretic alpha 1-globulin pattern of serum in alpha 1-antitrypsin deficiency. *Scandinavian J Clin & Lab Investigation*. 15:132-140.

Perlmutter, DH. 1995. Clinical manifestations of alpha 1-antitrypsin deficiency. *Gastroenterology Clin of No Amer*. (Mar) 24, 1:27-43.

Singer et al. 1999. Quality end-of-life care. *JAMA*. (Jan) 231, 2:163-168.

Stoller, JK. 1997. Clinical features and natural history of severe alpha 1-antitrypsin deficiency. *Chest*. 111:123S-128S.

Stoller, JK, P Smith, P Yang, and J Spray. 1994. Physical and social impact of alpha 1-antitrypsin deficiency: results of a survey. *Cleveland Clin J Med*. Nov-Dec: 461-467.

Trulock, EP. 1996. Lung transplantation for alpha 1-antitrypsin deficiency emphysema. *Chest* Suppl: *Alpha 1-antitrypsin: a world view*. 284S-294S.

21

Hospice Care and COPD

Harold Haley, MD

With an aging population and increased recognition of the value of hospice care for other than cancer patients, it can be expected that more patients with chronic obstructive pulmonary disease (COPD) will come to hospice, as both inpatient and outpatient. Present experience is that hospices have patients with COPD alone, with accompanying congestive heart failure (CHF), with lung cancer, with infections (especially pneumonias), or with various more nonspecific comorbidities such as diabetes mellitus or stroke. This chapter will touch on all of these.

For COPD patients, the purpose of hospice is to provide comfort and care and maximize the quality of life near its end. The majority of hospice patients are covered by the Medicare benefit, which is based on an expected duration of life of 6 months or less. To establish this, Medicare uses standards based on National Hospice Association Guidelines. HMOs and insurance carriers often use the same standards. With other than cancer patients, 6-month prognostic estimates are difficult. Benefits may go on longer, but continuing deterioration must be well documented. According to the Hospice Medical Policy Manual of Wellmark, Inc., a federal intermediary and carrier:

> Patients will be considered to be in the terminal stages of pulmonary disease (life expectancy of six months or less) if they meet the following criteria:
> 1. Severe chronic lung disease as documented by both a and b;
>   a. Disabling dyspnea at rest, poorly or unresponsive to bronchodilators, resulting in decreased functional capacity, eg, bed to chair existence, fatigue, and cough. (Documentation of Forced Expiratory Volume in One Second [FEV_1], after bronchodilator, less than 30% of predicted is objective evidence for disabling dyspnea, but it is not necessary to obtain.)
>   b. Progression of end stage pulmonary disease, as evidenced by increasing visits to the emergency department or hospitalizations for pulmonary infections and/or respiratory failure or increasing physician home visits prior to initial certification. (Documentation of serial decrease of FEV_1 below 30% is objective evidence for disease progression, but is not necessary to obtain.)

2. Hypoxemia at rest on room air, as evidence by Po_2 of less than 55 mm Hg or oxygen saturation of 88% on supplemental oxygen determined either by arterial blood gases or oxygen saturation monitors (these values may be obtained from recent hospital records) or hypercapnia, as evidenced by Pco_2 above 50 mm Hg (this value may be obtained from recent [within 3 months] hospital records).

3. Right Heart Failure secondary to pulmonary disease (cor pulmonale) (eg, not secondary to left heart disease or valvulopathy).

These three must be present. Documentation of unintentional progressive weight loss of greater than 10% of body weight over the preceding six months and/or resting tachycardia greater than 100/min lends support.

Patients with both COPD and CHF are frequently seen in hospice. Each condition makes the other worse. Determination of which condition is causing particular symptoms is difficult and treatments for each are different, are overlapping, and may cause problems with the other condition. For example, fluid accumulation in CHF is treated by diuretics, which if overused can cause dehydration, which can make the patient's COPD cough worse. According to Wellmark's *Hospice Medical Policy Manual*:

Recognizing that the determination of life expectancy during the course of terminal illness is difficult, this intermediary has established medical criteria for determining prognosis for non-cancer diagnoses. These criteria form a reasonable approach to the determination of the expectancy based on available research, and may be revised as more research is available. Skillful palliation in patients with end stage heart disease, including judicious use of diuretics and vasodilators, particularly angiotensin-converting enzyme (ACE) inhibitors, may promote survival for long periods with extremely severe symptoms. Conversely, some patients with advanced coronary disease may die suddenly and unexpectedly from acute ventricular arrhythmias. Coverage of hospice care for patients not meeting the criteria in this policy may be denied. However, some patients may not meet the criteria, but still be appropriate for hospice care, because of other comorbidities or rapid decline. Coverage for these patients may be approved on an individual consideration basis....

Patients will be considered to be in the terminal stage of heart disease (life expectancy of six months or less) if they meet the following criteria. (1 and 2 must be present. Factors from 3 will add supporting documentation.)

1. At the time of initial certification or recertification for hospice, the patient is or has been already optimally treated for congestive heart failure with diuretics and vasodilators, usually including ACE inhibitors, or have angina pectoris at rest which is resistant to intensive medical therapy or are patients who are either not candidates for revascularization procedures or decline these procedures. (Optimally treated means that patients who are not on vasodilators have a medical reason for refusing these drugs, eg, hypotension or renal disease.)

2. The patient is classified as New York Heart Association Class IV and has significant symptoms of recurrent congestive heart failure at rest. (Class IV patients with heart disease have an inability to carry on any physical activity without discomfort. Symptoms of heart failure or of the anginal syndrome may be present even at rest. If any physical activity is undertaken, discomfort is increased.) Significant congestive heart failure may be documented by an ejection fraction of 20%, but is not required if not already available....

4. Documentation of the following factors will support but is not required to establish eligibility for hospice care:
   a. Treatment resistant symptomatic supraventricular or ventricular arrhythmias;
   b. History of cardiac arrest or resuscitation;
   c. History of unexplained syncope;
   d. Brain embolism of cardiac origin;
   e. Concomitant HIV disease.

Hospice provides medical and social care for COPD patients, with symptom relief and patient comfort being primary concerns. Dyspnea (or breathlessness) is the most common symptom and can be devastating to patients and cause extreme feelings of helplessness in caregivers. This is often associated with weakness because of the breathlessness brought on by even the slightest exertion. Hospice staff administer, supervise, and monitor the prescribed treatments, such as oxygen, bronchodilators, and opiates. Morphine relieves much dyspnea. Dosages can be titrated to limit any respiratory depression. Anxiety and agitation are frequent and require treatment. Pain and discomfort are often present: there may be chest or rib pain, or body or bone pain, possibly related to prolonged immobilization and fear of moving because of breathlessness. There may be gastrointestinal symptoms, often related to various medications. If the patient also has right or biventricular heart disease, these may require treatment. Such treatments can complicate COPD treatment. Diuretic therapy can lead to dehydration, which can affect secretions and respiratory symptoms. With all of these multiple clinical problems, the physician must develop a treatment plan specifically for the individual patient. Hospice staff can administer treatments, educate caregivers about medications and other treatments, monitor progress, and communicate professionally with the physician.

Part of providing good care is giving all care that will alleviate symptoms, while minimizing procedures and medications that do not affect the current care and comfort. On the all-too-long medication lists that patients come with, we see such things as anti-lipid drugs with a long-range intent that does not seem appropriate at the end of life. This is part of monitoring.

Hospice staff have other functions besides symptom relief. Monitoring change in the patient's condition and adjusting therapies to meet needs as they develop are important. Another important function is maximizing the environment to meet patient needs, including beds, bathroom, and temperature.

Relationships with family members and other caregivers are critical. Patients and families need much education concerning the disease process, prognosis, what can be expected to happen, what caregivers should watch for, and what procedures they can perform, as well as answers to the questions that will inevitably come up. Hospice does not provide 24-hour care in the home, but staff is on call all day, all night, and weekends. The middle-of-the-night events, which may or may not be true emergencies, cause much anxiety in caregivers, resulting in phone calls to hospice staff who may be able to alleviate the problem on the telephone. Often, however, these calls result in the nurse on call going to the patient's home.

Seriously ill patients and their families face difficult problems in areas that they do not always understand, such as legal and financial matters and in dealings with government and insurance companies. Hospice staff, especially social workers, understand these types of problems and help patients and families survive in these jungles.

Volunteers also serve an important role, performing many helpful functions. These include providing transportation to the doctor's office or elsewhere and being in the home with the patient to allow the caregiver to go the store, church, or his or her own doctor, or just to get away for a while. When someone is very ill and dying, fear of being alone can be overwhelming; hospice volunteers help by their presence.

Having said all these things, it must be added that good palliative hospice care may very well improve the patient's condition and slow down clinical deterioration. With deterioration slowing, the patient may be saved from emergency room visits and hospitalizations. We have documented fewer such episodes than patients had prior to hospice. Note that this improvement may extend the 6-month period, requiring strong drive for recertification.

Perhaps the most important thing that hospice staff can give patients is time, while being helpful, communicative, and caring.

22

Hospice Care for Patients With Advanced COPD

Janet L. Abrahm, MD, FACP

History of the Modern Hospice Movement

The modern hospice movement began in Great Britain, Canada, and the United States in the late 1960s and early 1970s, with the founding of hospices offering both in-home and inpatient services. St. Christopher's Hospice, the first such hospice, was established in London in 1967. Dame Cicely Saunders, its founding medical director, introduced its emphasis on research to improve the care of the dying: "In the hospice movement we continue to be concerned both with the sophisticated science of our treatments and with the art of our caring, bringing competence alongside compassion" (Saunders 1981).

The hospice movement in the United States spread in the late 1970s. The movement's growth, supported almost entirely by donations, coincided with the publication and popularity of *On Death and Dying* by Dr. Elisabeth Kubler-Ross in 1975 (Fulton 1981). Dying Americans and those who cared for them began to seek a better, less technological death at home, and hospice helped make that wish a reality (Mor 1988). Hospices worked to counter an active euthanasia movement, as well as "the loneliness, isolation, lack of family involvement and unrelieved pain that came to be synonymous with individuals dying in acute care hospitals" (Fulton 1981). In 1977, the National Hospice Organization (NHO) was established as a multidisciplinary organization of hospice personnel, and in 1988, the American Academy of Hospice and Palliative Medicine was founded (then called the Academy of Hospice Physicians), its mission being to bring together physicians dedicated to promoting quality hospice/palliative care through medical education, research, and training. In 1997, the NHO estimated that there were almost 3000 operational hospice programs in the United States, which served approximately 450,000 patients per year, or about 17% of all patients who die each year (Kinzbrunner 1998; Committee on Care at the End of Life 1997).

Hospices must be accredited and certified, and some states require hospices to be licensed and inspected. The Joint Commission on Accreditation of Healthcare Organizations (JCAHO) accredits hospices within the category of home care organizations; it has no specific hospice accreditation standards (Donaldson 1998). The Health Care Financing Administration accepts JCAHO accreditation as fulfilling the Conditions of Participation for Medicare Hospice Programs. The NHO has also prepared a quality statement titled *Standards of a Hospice Program of Care* (1993) that includes stipulated guidelines for hospice quality assessment programs.

The Hospice Philosophy

Hospice seeks neither to prolong life nor to hasten death. The focus of care is to provide patients and families with comfort and dignity and to enhance the quality of the remaining life. Hospice caregivers help patients and families identify and realize their remaining hopes and goals. Hospice care includes physical, social, psychological/emotional, and spiritual dimensions, as described below. In the United States, most hospice care takes place in the home, although hospice is increasingly involved in the care of inpatients and of nursing home residents. Hospice also prepares families for their loss and offers continued assistance after death through bereavement programs.

Hospice views the time remaining to patients as very active, filled with the many goals that patients and their families wish to accomplish before death. A patient with unrelieved physical, psychological, or spiritual suffering has neither the energy nor the presence of mind to pursue these tasks. The role of the hospice team is much like that of Michelangelo, who could see his future work of art in the block of marble. His challenge was to free the statue from the stone. Michelangelo's statues of unfinished slaves (Academy Museum in Florence, Italy), in fact, seem to be striving to complete their liberation. If hospice patients are to travel, visit with family, prepare a legacy, or quietly reflect or pray as they work to make sense of their life stories, similar energy must be used to eliminate the unnecessary and to practice the art of expert palliative care.

Clinical Care Provided

Hospice can be an enormous source of comfort to families and professional caregivers, particularly for those who have never witnessed a "natural" death. The team members have experience, can explain what is likely to happen, and can provide expert symptom management during the last days and hours.

Early referral is very beneficial. After 1 or 2 months together, hospice workers have an enhanced understanding of the patient's and family's needs and are effective at providing help during the last days. Staff try to ensure that the family of the patient is comfortable with the choices that have been made about the patient's care and minimize any guilt family members may feel about these choices when the patient dies.

Levels of Care

Hospices provide a continuum of care, from home to an inpatient setting. While most patients are cared for in their homes, as stated in the 1993 Federal Regulations, all Medicare-certified hospices are required to provide four levels of care: routine, continuous, respite, and inpatient.

Routine care services are offered 24 hours a day, 7 days a week. A registered nurse is on call to respond to patient or family needs and makes home visits when necessary. Services include home nursing (at least weekly but more often as required); occupational, speech, or physical therapy; and home health aide and social services as required. The hospice team chaplain also offers home visits or coordinated care with the patient's own clergy. Volunteers, who are usually available 2 to 4 hours a week, help families in nonclinical areas. A hospice medical director works with the team and the patient's primary physician to optimize symptom management.

Continuous home care is provided for patients who require continuous symptom management and for whom the home care setting remains appropriate. Patients with unrelieved cough, dyspnea, pain, or delirium, for example, can receive 24-hour nursing and home health aide services until the problem is brought under control. Home visits from a hospice medical director can also be provided.

Respite care is provided by a community skilled or intermediate nursing facility with which the hospice has a contract. The nursing care facility provides all the services necessary for patient comfort. The goal of respite care is to provide a rest for the caregiver or to remove the patient to an adequate facility when the home is temporarily inadequate to meet the patient's care needs. The number of days for respite care varies with the type of insurance, but patients eligible for the Medicare Hospice Benefit (explained in detail later in this chapter) are entitled to 5 days per month.

Hospice patients rarely require inpatient care, and fewer than 1% die in hospitals. But if a patient's symptoms cannot be controlled at home, even with continuous care, the patient can be hospitalized under the Medicare Hospice Benefit. The hospice team is responsible for the plan of care, just as they were in the patient's home, and team members visit the patient as they would an outpatient. A hospice medical director is available to provide consultation for symptom management, but the referring physician remains the primary physician and may bill for his/her services under Medicare Part B. Orders for the patient's care are written by inpatient unit personnel, and inpatient staff provide the care. The per diem allotted by Medicare for an inpatient on hospice is approximately $400.

Occasionally, hospice patients require hospital admission for reasons unrelated to the primary diagnosis. A patient with advanced chronic obstructive pulmonary disease (COPD) may fall and break a hip. That patient would be admitted, covered under Medicare Part B, and would not be disenrolled from hospice.

Roles of Team Members

Hospice patients are cared for by medically directed, interdisciplinary teams that include the attending physician, the hospice medical director, a nursing director of patient services, an office administrator, a nurse, a social worker, home health aides, a chaplain, and volunteers. Bereavement counselors become involved after the patient's death but are available to family members before death, if needed. The core team can also request additional consultations from physicians, registered dietitians, and occupational, speech, or physical therapists.

The primary nurse is responsible for assessment and management of the patient's physical and often psychological distress, visiting usually twice weekly, but more often as needed. She or he also provides education about the disease and the recommended treatments, including practical instruction in how the family can help with toileting, feeding, massage, and the administering of medications.

As death approaches, the primary nurse provides suggestions for answering patient questions. When requested or when appropriate, she or he reviews the dying process and furnishes written materials that explain how the family or the personnel in inpatient or long-term care facilities can determine that death is imminent. The primary nurse also describes the signs and symptoms of dying, instructs family in emergency procedures, and is available for support while the patient dies.

The social worker assesses the social and financial needs of the dying patient and his or her family and identifies those who are at risk for a particularly painful bereavement period. Social workers offer support and family counseling and, often working with the chaplain, try to facilitate any needed family reconciliation. They engage the patient and family in advance care and funeral planning if the patient and family so desire; advise on the desirability of living wills and durable powers of attorney and assist in their execution if requested; provide applications for financial aid or waivers; and help identify financing for additional home health care. They assist patients in making plans for their survivors (eg, guardianship for children) and in completing life reviews.

Chaplains provide support both for the traditionally religious and for those who have spiritual or existential sources of distress (eg, loss of hope, loss of connection or love, a need for forgiveness or to forgive, a need to identify the meaning of their lives).

Volunteers do any number of tasks, depending on the family's needs. Services include sitting with the patient to enable the caregiver to go to church, doing the shopping, driving the patient or caregiver to doctor appointments, or picking up supplies. Volunteers provide phone support, and they are especially vital for hospice patients who live alone.

Bereavement counselors may provide support for family members experiencing "anticipatory grief" prior to a patient's death and routinely communicate with the bereaved for the first year after the death. Survivors receive letters containing advice, and they may be invited to memorial services and to participate in drop-in support groups or groups designed to meet special needs (eg, parents who have lost young children, teenagers who have lost a parent).

Medications/Treatments Provided

Hospice provides 95% of the cost of prescription drugs related to a terminal diagnosis and necessary for palliative treatment (and many hospices waive the other 5% if there is no insurance coverage). Hospice provides all durable medical equipment, supplies, and oxygen for needs related to the terminal diagnosis; laboratory and diagnostic procedures related to the terminal diagnosis; and transportation when medically necessary for changes in the patient's level of care.

While maximizing a patient's quality of life is a central goal of hospice, it is not always possible for a patient to be both comfortable and awake and interactive. Fewer than 5% of hospice patients will fall into this category, but those who suffer from refractory pain, cough, dyspnea, or delirium, must be treated to the point of sedation before the symptom abates. Using appropriate combinations of opioids, anticholinergics (such as scopolamine or hyoscyamine [Levsin SL®]), and sedatives such as benzodiazepines or barbiturates, with the rare addition of anesthetics such as propofol or ketamine, patients can be sedated to what appears to be a comfortable level. Intravenous hydration or enteral or parenteral nutrition can be provided if it meets the goals set by the patient, his or her family, and the hospice team. (They are rarely used in imminently dying patients whether or not they are sedated because, as McCann et al (1994) found, these patients are rarely suffering from hunger or thirst.) When opioids and sedatives are employed, sedation can be accomplished using the continuous care option in the patient's home; administration of anesthetics requires hospitalization.

Common Misconceptions

- *Patients enrolling in hospice must choose not to be resuscitated.*
  Patients do not have to relinquish the right to be resuscitated to enroll in hospice. Hospices will inform patients and families that staff members will not perform the resuscitation themselves, but will call 911 if requested to do so. Hospice personnel do assist patients and their families in advance care planning and inform patients' physicians of the status of these discussions. Most commonly, following a thorough explanation of the implications by hospice personnel, patients elect not to be resuscitated.

- *Patients enrolled in hospice lose their primary physicians.*
  Referring attending physicians continue to direct and approve patient care, from initial certification of terminal prognosis to the medication and durable medical equipment orders, approving the frequency of home health aide visits and consultations, and certifying the resuscitation status. (If patients require either inpatient hospice admission for symptom control or routine admission for diagnoses unrelated to the terminal illness, physicians may bill Medicare under Part B for any visits.)

- *Hospices would rather enroll cancer patients than patients with non-malignant diagnoses.*
  In the past, hospices traditionally did enroll a larger proportion of cancer patients than noncancer patients because they were referred more often, probably because physicians felt more certain the cancer patients would not exceed the "6 month" prognosis requirement of the Medicare Hospice Benefit. The NHO, however, developed guidelines for noncancer diagnoses to encourage referrals of patients with other conditions. Some patients who would otherwise be eligible for hospice, though, may not be enrolled because of the cost of some of the medications or treatments that would be required for palliation. It may not be possible, for example, for a small hospice to offer care to a patient with refractory congestive heart failure who requires a daily intravenous inotrope costing more than $500 a day for the drug alone when the Medicare per diem is $100.

- *Hospice patients cannot be hospitalized and remain enrolled in hospice.*
  Any hospice patient can be admitted to an acute, inpatient level of care if it is needed to control a distressing symptom. Hospices are required to offer this level of care. Some hospices work with designated inpatient palliative care units, some contract with acute care hospitals for beds, and others have their own inpatient facilities in which they can deliver the intensity of care required.

- *Hospice patients cannot participate in research projects while enrolled in hospice.*
  A hospice patient can participate in a research project, as long as the project is consistent with the mission of hospice. Funding for palliative care and end-of-life research is increasing and hospice patients will be sought to participate as researchers strive to learn more about the dying process, how to assess and alleviate sources of suffering, and how to change the health care delivery system to provide more uniform access to care for this population.

- *Hospice nursing personnel do not provide sophisticated care.*
  Hospice personnel provide expert palliative care. They do not simply hold patients' hands, place cool washcloths on their foreheads, and change linens. The palliative care they deliver requires astute assessment and expert intervention tailored to patient and family goals. For patients with advanced obstructive lung disease, this includes pharmacologic and nonpharmacologic (eg, noninvasive nocturnal ventilation, oxygen, air-conditioning, fans) treatments of common disorders, such as dyspnea, cough, right heart failure, fatigue, pain, insomnia, anxiety, and depression. Tube feedings, intravenous hydration, or intravenous medications to control symptoms may also be provided depending on the clinical status of the patient.

- *Patients can "use up" their hospice eligibility, so it is important not to enroll too soon.*
  Patients who live longer than 6 months will continue to receive services, as long as they continue to meet the eligibility criteria for hospice care. They are initially certified for 3 months of service, after which their physicians and the hospice medical director are asked to recertify them for another 3-month period. After that, recertification can take place indefinitely, at 2-month intervals. In addition, patients who chose to revoke the hospice benefit to seek life-prolonging therapies may choose to re-enroll if their goals change.

- *Patients must have a live-in caregiver to enroll in hospice.*
  Many hospices care for "live-alone" patients, employing special protocols to enhance their safety (Bly 1994). Medical alert devices worn around the neck, "lock-boxes" to provide access in an emergency, and daily patient contact are some of the measures used. Patients are also strongly encouraged to work with the social workers to develop a plan for nursing home placement if they become too debilitated to continue at home alone.

The Medicare Hospice Benefit

The Medicare Hospice Benefit was established in 1982 as part of the Tax Equity and Fiscal Responsibility Act (Section 122). Then, as now, the attending physician and the hospice medical director were both required to certify that the patient was terminally ill, with a prognosis of 6 months or less if the disease were to follow its usual course, before the patient would be eligible for the Medicare Hospice Benefit. In addition to the Medicare benefit, Medicaid, private insurers, and health maintenance organizations all offer some form of hospice benefit (Committee on Care 1997). The general programs are similar, but the availability of inpatient hospice, the number of respite days, and the total spending cap available for each patient vary. Hospice nurses and social workers identify and access all programs that might provide a patient or family benefit and work with primary physicians and hospice medical directors to gain approval for them.

A report by the Institute of Medicine could not conclude whether hospice as currently regulated and funded is or is not cost-effective and concludes that "hospice programs should be promoted on non-economic grounds related to their emphasis on medical and non-medical care goals, attention to families and others close to their patient, provision for non-medical supportive services ... and similar features" (Committee on Care 1997). Meier et al (1997) suggest that "although the cost would depend on the timing of hospice referral, hospice care is less expensive (on average) than traditional medical care."

Admission Criteria

Traditionally, most of the patients referred for hospice care had a diagnosis of cancer (NHO 1991). The likely reason was the emphasis placed by the enabling legislation on the requirement that the physician certify a 6-month prognosis. While patients with refractory congestive heart failure or advanced COPD can be certified as having a terminal illness, actual time of death is much more difficult to predict. In 1995, committees of experts from the NHO were convened to create criteria that would help physicians identify patients with nonmalignant terminal illnesses who would qualify for hospice. Stuart et al (1996) published expanded NHO guidelines, and in 1997, the Health Care Financing Administration codified the guidelines into auditable criteria by which to judge appropriateness of hospice referral. Despite protestations from the original guideline developers, these remain, with some emendation from hospice experts, the Local Medical Review Policies of the Medicare fiscal intermediaries.

Criteria for advanced lung disease were last modified in June 1998 (Wellmark 1998). In full, they read:

> Patients will be considered to be in the terminal stage of pulmonary disease (life expectancy of six months or less) if they meet the following criteria. The criteria refer to patients with various forms of advanced pulmonary disease who eventually follow a final common pathway for end stage pulmonary disease (1, 2, and 3 must be present. Documentation of 4 or 5 will lend supporting documentation.):
>
> 1. Severe chronic lung disease as documented by both a. and b.:
>   a. Disabling dyspnea at rest, poorly or unresponsive to bronchodilators, resulting in decreased functional capacity, eg bed to chair existence, fatigue, and cough. (Documentation of Forced Expiratory Volume in one second [FEV_1], after bronchodilator less than 30% of predicted is objective evidence for disabling dyspnea, but is not necessary to obtain.)
>   b. Progression of end stage pulmonary disease, as evidenced by increasing visits to the emergency department or hospitalizations for

pulmonary infections and/or respiratory failure or increasing physician home visits prior to initial certification. (Documentation of serial decrease of FEV_1 > 40 ml/yr is objective evidence for disease progression, but is not necessary to obtain.)

2. Hypoxemia at rest on room air, as evidenced by PO_2 = 55 mm Hg or oxygen saturation < 88% on supplemental oxygen determined either by arterial blood gases or oxygen saturation monitors (these values may be obtained from recent hospital records), or hypercapnea, as evidenced by PCO_2 > 50 mm Hg (this value may be obtained from recent [within 3 months] hospital records).

3. Right heart failure secondary to pulmonary disease (Cor pulmonale) (eg not secondary to left heart disease or valvulopathy).

4. Unintentional progressive weight loss of greater than 10% of body weight over the preceding six months.

5. Resting tachycardia > 100/min.

Documentation: Documentation certifying terminal status must contain enough information to confirm terminal status upon review. Documentation meeting the above criteria would meet this requirement. If the patient does not meet the above criteria, yet is deemed appropriate for hospice care, sufficient documentation of the patient's condition that justifies terminal status, in the absence of meeting the above criteria, would be necessary. Documentation might include comorbidities, rapid decline in physical or functional status in spite of appropriate treatment, or symptom severity that with reasonable reliability is consistent with a life span prognosis of six months or less.

Implementation

In 1995, the Office of the Inspector General began audits for fraud and abuse in nursing homes, home health agencies, suppliers of durable medical equipment, and hospices, looking especially for ineligible patients and hospices with high proportions of patients who exceeded the 6-month length of stay. Virtually none of the institutions was found guilty of fraud or abuse, but the fear of such an accusation caused a number of hospices to adhere more strictly to the admission criteria and many doctors to delay referrals until certain of the prognosis. As reported by Christakis et al (1996), in 1990 the median time of survival after hospice admission was approximately 1 month, which may now be less than 3 weeks (Kinzbrunner 1998). In one large for-profit hospice, for example, the average length of stay for cancer patients dropped from 59 days in the 1993-1994 academic year to 43 days in the 1997-1998 academic year; median stays in the same periods dropped from 19 to 17 days (Kinzbrunner 1999). Currently, hospices are still undergoing aggressive focused audits.

Financial Considerations

The Medicare Hospice Benefit is a managed care, capitated reimbursement program that reimburses hospices on a per diem basis, based on each patient's level of care (approximately $100 per day for routine or respite care and $400 per day for inpatient acute care). Medicaid, private insurance, and health maintenance providers reimburse hospices at various rates, and with the last, services must be approved through the plan's case manager. Most hospices therefore must secure additional funding from grants and private donations to pay for the mandated services. A patient, or his or her designated power of attorney, elects hospice to provide for all of the palliative care required during the terminal illness. Medical needs that are unrelated to the terminal illness remain covered by Medicare Part A or Part B, as appropriate.

Providing Hospice in Skilled Nursing Facilities

In skilled nursing facilities, patients receive Medicare benefits for skilled care and cannot retain these and enroll in the Medicare Hospice Benefit. Since 1989, Medicaid patients and those who pay for their own care in nursing homes have been eligible to enroll in hospice (Miller 1998). The Medicaid payment for room and board is assigned to the hospice, and the hospice, in turn, reimburses the nursing home for the patient's room and board and any additional costs related to the care and treatment of the terminal illness. Hospice can provide significant additional resources, such as health aides and chaplain services. Further, since nursing home staff often serve as a patient's surrogate family, hospice also tries to meet staff needs, including counseling for anticipatory grief and bereavement.

Providing Aggressive Palliation

Given the reimbursement schedule, aggressive palliation is often prohibitively expensive for small to medium-sized hospices. Certain expensive radiation therapies and chemotherapeutic or hematopoietic agents are purely palliative; other therapies, however, provide palliation and also extend life. These might include dialysis for a patient with renal failure from refractory multiple myeloma; inotrope infusions for patients in severe congestive heart failure; or pamidronate for a patient with hypercalcemia and bone pain. A hospice must decide which treatments are consistent with its philosophy and which it can afford.

Limitations of Current Hospice Model

Admission Criteria

Clearly, for patients with COPD, the admission criteria are a significant barrier to early hospice referral. Prospective studies of other prognostic models may provide better criteria. If, despite such efforts, the 6-month standard leaves substantial numbers of such patients unserved by appropriate end-of-life care, models designated to identify and care for COPD patients in the last few years of life may be the answer.

Professional Barriers

In the current medical culture, it is very difficult to refer appropriate patients to hospice at the appropriate time. Physicians are rarely informed about how much there is to offer patients whose disease is refractory to life-prolonging therapy. Also, as Meier and colleagues (1997) state, "clinicians may ... feel inadequate, guilty, or sad when curative therapies or treatment that prolong life have been exhausted, and assume that there is 'nothing left to do.' " Difficulty also exists in identifying who among the severely ill is actually dying and who among these has executed an advance directive that might induce a hospice referral (Muller 1988, Kaufman 1998). Physicians may be overly optimistic about prognosis, or may fear censure if they refer patients who live longer than 6 months.

Patient/Family Barriers

Generally, American patients seem very resistant to accepting a terminal prognosis. The Institute of Medicine, for example, noted "a deeply ingrained public philosophy of individualism, and a general American unwillingness to accept limits—including aging and death" (Committee on Care 1997). Daniel Callahan (1995) also stated that Americans have "an unwillingness to let nature take its course," which can lead to "death in a technological cocoon." When asked where they would want to die of a terminal illness, 90% of Americans said they would want to die at home, but only 20% actually do die at home and 40% to 60% die in hospitals (Committee on Care 1997, Meier 1997). Perhaps this is because over 60% stated they would still seek curative therapy (Committee on Care 1997). To enroll in hospice, patients must acknowledge their 6-month prognosis, relinquish further curative therapy, and give informed consent. These requirements may be serious obstacles to hospice enrollment (Kinzbrunner 1998).

Hospice coverage is offered by only 80% of large- and medium-sized employers and hospice coverage for those not eligible for Medicare or Medicaid varies greatly in terms of what services and providers are covered and with what limitations (eg, exclusions for preexisting conditions) (Committee on Care 1997).

Further, in hospice, 80% of the patient's care must, by law, take place at his or her home. While hospice provides some help, the majority of the patient's care must be provided by family or friends or by privately paid professional caregivers, so some patients will not be able to stay at home even with the maximum help hospice personnel and volunteers can offer.

Benefits of Hospice Integration Into Inpatient and Outpatient Settings

Hospice is a natural partner to efforts directed at improving symptom control, other aspects of quality of life, advance care planning, and bereavement services to families.

Whenever patients are admitted to inpatient hospice, the hospice personnel who visit the patient to implement the plan of care are superb resources to the unit care team and can provide services relating to the physical, psychological, and spiritual comfort to patients at the end of life and to their families. In addition, to be able to reach more dying patients and their families, community hospices are increasingly participating in other roles in traditional care settings. Some hospices help to staff inpatient palliative care teams that also identify patients suitable for hospice. Others send teams into outpatient clinics at cancer centers to identify and help resolve palliative care needs. Many have separate skilled nursing services staffed by hospice-trained nurses and social workers, who care for homebound terminally ill patients with skilled care needs who do not wish to enroll in hospice. By exploring such innovative partnerships, clinicians caring for patients with advanced COPD may be able to greatly enhance the quality of life for patients and their families.

Equally important, hospice can help unit staff cope both intellectually and emotionally with their losses. Medical students and resident physicians are particularly vulnerable to feelings of guilt, inadequacy, and loss following the deaths of patients they have cared for. They may carry these unresolved feelings with them into their professional careers and not be aware of the typical physical, psychological, and spiritual manifestations of their grief or of effective coping strategies. In units in which death is a frequent occurrence, regular meetings with hospice-trained bereavement experts may be of significant benefit to developing physicians.

In his 1996 address to medical students entering the University of California-San Francisco, Dr. Lloyd Holly Smith said:

> We have all been patients or we shall be in our time. What do patients want? Patients want to be listened to so that their fears can be fully expressed. They want to be considered as unique individuals of dignity and worth, especially during the course of a degrading or frightening illness.

They certainly want the best of modern medical science to be brought to bear upon their problems, but in the human context of personal interactions and empathy.

This is the area in which hospice excels and this is what it has to offer, not only to the dying and their families, but to all those who care for them.

References

42 Codes of Federal Regulations, Pt 418. 1993. Medicare Hospice Regulations.

Bly, J and PD Kissick. 1994. Hospice care for persons living alone. Evaluation of demonstration program sponsored by Wissahickon Hospice: final report.

Bulkin, W and H Lukashok. 1988. Rx for dying: the case for hospice. *N Eng J Med.* 318:376-378.

Callahan, D. 1995. Frustrated mastery: the cultural context of death in America. *West J Med.* 163:226-230.

Committee on Care at the End of Life, Institute of Medicine. 1997. The health care system and the dying patient. In *Approaching Death, Improving Care at the End of Life*, eds. MJ Field and CK Cassel, 87-121. Washington, DC: National Academy Press.

————. 1997. Financial and economic issues in end-of-life care. In *Approaching Death, Improving Care at the End of Life*, eds. MJ Field and CK Cassel, 154-187. Washington, DC: National Academy Press.

————. 1997. A profile of death and dying in America. In *Approaching Death, Improving Care at the End of Life*, eds. MJ Field and CK Cassel, 33-49. Washington, DC: National Academy Press.

Donaldson, MS and MJ Field. 1998. Measuring quality of care at the end of life. *Arch Int Med.* 158:121-128.

Federal Registry DHEW Health Care Financing Administration. Dec 16, 1983. *Medicare Program; Hospice Care; Final Rule.* Part VII.

Fulton, R and G Owen. 1981. Hospice in America; from principle to practice. In *Hospice: The Living Idea*, eds. C Saunders, DH Summers, and N Teller, 9-18. Philadelphia, PA: WB Saunders, Co.

Gallup, GH. 1997. Spiritual beliefs and the dying process: a report on a national survey conducted for the Nathan Cummings Foundation and Fetzer Institute. (Oct) Princeton, NJ: The George H Gallup International Institute.

Kaufman, SR. 1998. Intensive care, old age, and the problem of death in America. *Gerontologist.* 38:715-725.

Kinzbrunner, BM. 1998. Hospice: 15 years and beyond in the care of the dying. *J Palliative Med.* 1:127-137.

————. 1999. Utilization of hospice services by terminally ill cancer patients. *Proc Amer Society of Clinical Oncology.* 18:577A.

McCann, RM, WJ Hall, and A Groth-Junker. 1994. Comfort care for terminally ill patients; the appropriate use of nutrition and hydration. *JAMA.* 272:1263-1266.

Meier, DE, RS Morrison, and CK Cassel. 1997. Improving palliative care. *Annals Int Med.* 127:225-230.

Miller, SC, V Mor, K Coppola, J Teno, L Laliberte, and AC Petrisek. 1998. The Medicare hospice benefit's influence on dying in nursing homes. *J Pall Med.* 1:367-376.

Mor, V, DS Greer, and R Kastenbaum, eds. 1988. *The Hospice Experiment*. Baltimore, MD: Johns Hopkins University Press.

Muller, JH and B Koenig. 1988. On the boundary of life and death: the definition of dying by medical residents. In *Biomedicine Examined*, eds. M Lock and D Gordon, 351-374. Boston: Kluwer.

National Hospice Organization. 1991. *Standards of a Hospice Program of Care*. Arlington, VA: National Hospice Organization.

Rhymes, J. 1990. Hospice care in America. *JAMA*. 264:369-372

Saunders, C. 1981. The founding philosophy. In *Hospice: The Living Idea*, eds. C Saunders, DBE, DH Summers, and N Teller, 4. Philadelphia: WB Saunders Co.

Rousseau, P, ed. 1998. *Academy Update*. 1:10

Stuart, B, S Connor, BM Kinzbrunner et al. 1996. *Medical Guidelines for Determining Prognosis in Selected Non-cancer Diseases*. 2nd ed. Arlington, VA: National Hospice Organization.

Wellmark, Inc. 1998. *Hospice Medical Policy Manual*.

23

Self-Help Groups and Members at Advanced Disease Stages

Daryl Holtz Isenberg, PhD, and Hannah L. Hedrick, PhD

> *If we don't have peace, it is because*
> *we have forgotten that we all belong to each other.*
> —Mother Theresa

In a 1989 study, psychiatrist David Spiegel reported the difference in survival rates between two groups of women with metastatic breast cancer. Those women who participated in weekly self-help group sessions lived an average of 36.6 months, while women who that did not participate in weekly sessions lived an average of 18 months. While not all studies of the impact of self-help group membership on survival report such dramatically increased survival rates, members and their families consistently report that the education, self-care techniques, and peer support provided by self-help groups enhance their ability to reduce stress and cope with the multiple challenges related to advanced disease stages.

Since the Foundation of Thanatology convened a 1989 conference on self-help and life-threatening illness, the authors of this chapter have been collecting information about self-help group structures and methodologies specifically designed to support members who are dying. We wondered, for example, if local groups organized to respond to the needs of people with diabetes recognized it as a life-threatening illness and had mechanisms to support members with end-stage problems. What national self-help organizations and their chapters were focusing on support at the end of life? What made it possible for them to do so? For groups not currently responding to the needs of members at the end of life, what would they need to help them do so?

In 1998, Daryl Isenberg, PhD, president of the Illinois Self-Help Coalition, began to address these issues in a pilot questionnaire directed to leaders of support groups for cancer, breast cancer, Huntington's disease, scleroderma, heart disease, chronic fatigue syndrome, manic depression, colitis and ileitis, ostomy, sarcoidosis, and multiple sclerosis. The results are described below. Support provided by self-help groups for dying members was also discussed in a panel Dr. Isenberg organized for a 1997 symposium on "The Other 74%: Non-Cancer Life-Threatening Diseases and

Their End-of-Life Components." The panel also included Audrey Gardner, PhD, executive director of the National Self-Help Clearinghouse, Arlette Lefebreve, MD, founder of Disability Online, Delores Gregory, past board vice president and area leader of Recovery, Inc., and Sandra Conroy, founder of the National Sarcoidosis Resource Center.

Although none of the groups represented by the panelists had specific guidelines for helping members at the end of life or as they were dying, the panelists believed that such guidelines and specific programs could have a profound effect. In the absence of such guidelines, the panelists were nonetheless able to describe the many ways in which the existing structure of each group supports members at all stages of a life-threatening illness. This chapter: (1) describes the types of assistance provided by self-help groups, (2) suggests some models for improving outreach at the end of life, (3) provides detailed instructions for supporting a fellow member in achieving a peaceful death, and (4) comments on the need for resources and training to improve the support that groups provide at the end of life.

Assistance Provided by Groups

Autonomous self-help groups for life-threatening illnesses, which are volunteer run, usually focus primarily on helping members and their families understand and adjust to the disease and on providing information about treatment and medication options. But self-help groups may also expand the types of support they provide, including advocacy activities. For example, 25 years ago, physicians strongly recommended that parents institutionalize children with Down syndrome. Newly formed groups for Down syndrome first dealt with the needs of new parents with infants. As those children have become teenagers and young adults, such organizations have expanded their single focus of assisting with adjustment and coping issues to now include advocating for health and educational services.

The authors assumed that self-help groups related to life-threatening issues followed the same developmental model of responding to emerging needs. In the 1998 pilot questionnaire, Dr. Isenberg asked the following questions about the end of life:

- Do people in later disease stages continue to receive help from the group at the end of life?
- How do people who lead groups and those in the group discuss the end of life?
- Is the organizational type or sponsor of the group linked to end-of-life (EOL) discussion and services?
- How do people who lead groups and those in the group affect discussions of the end of life?
- Is the organizational type or sponsor of the group linked to EOL discussion?

From mid July to mid August 1999, a 3-page pilot questionnaire was sent to self-help group program coordinators, or to local chapters of national organizations if those organizations did not operate groups. Twenty-five groups were found to be either single national organizations or national chapters, and 7 autonomous local groups were selected. The national organizations that did not operate groups sent local chapter lists from which one or more were chosen throughout the United States. After contacting each organization we intended to survey, we sent out 35 questionnaires. Of these, two local chapters—National Ataxia Foundation and the Bronx Candlelighters Foundation—were no longer in service. Four national organizations related to advanced disease stages—Batten's Disease in San Francisco, Dysautonomia Foundation in New York, Children's Brain Tumor Foundation in New York, and Ronald McDonald House in New York—did not sponsor peer meetings for members; instead, they concentrated on advocacy, fundraising, or respite programs. Of the 35 questionnaires sent, 17 (nearly 50%) filled out the questionnaire.

Questionnaire Responses

There was considerable variation in the ways in which groups provided EOL assistance, depending to a certain extent on whether the group was related to a life-threatening illness, to a chronic and progressive illness, or to cognitive and emotional impairments. Some groups were more open than others to exploring materials and programs focusing on issues related to death and dying.

When questioned about what services were supplied in addition to meetings, the responses given most frequently were newsletters, educational material, and between-meeting visits. In addition, Huntington Disease groups offered counseling, case management, placement in long-term care, referrals, community presentations, and educational classes. Parkinson disease groups offered advocacy, summer camp, hotline services, conferences, exercise programs, social events, and assistive equipment. Cancer groups offer alternative health classes, summer camp, social events, advocacy, group leadership training, and financial assistance.

Answers to the question of what services groups would like to provide for members at the end of their lives included peer counseling, fellowship, visits, emotional and spiritual support, help with referral to hospice, respite for caregivers, transportation, and legal issues.

During conversation around the question "What else would you like us to consider about this topic?" respondents indicated they would like attention paid to unresolved grief among board and staff, assistance with helping professionals become more comfortable with the topic of death and dying, educational resources to help people become more open in sharing their own experiences, and more formal integration of complementary modalities during end of life care, including massage, energetic approaches, healing touch, and Reiki.

In answer to the question of whether members discuss taking charge of medical decisions, such as humane advance directives and where they would prefer to die, 12 (71%) reported that they do provide opportunities for such discussions, 1 respondent reported that the group does not discuss the topic, and 4 groups did not answer the question. Seventy-six percent provide opportunities for members to discuss relationship reconciliation as death approaches and to discuss regrets and what was meaningful in life. Eighty-two percent provide a forum for discussing spiritual and religious concepts about death. Only 10 groups (59%) reported providing opportunities for members to discuss grief and loss at the end of life, usually in special meetings or educational programs.

In 76% of the groups, people in the later disease stages continued to receive group services. Sixty-four percent reported knowledge of group members responding informally to fellow members facing the end of life, through visits at home or in the hospital or by coordinating food services. Only 7 groups (41%) reported using the Internet to provide support to the dying person and family.

When asked what kinds of information dissemination formats they would find most helpful, 59% indicated that they would welcome handouts, while 41% felt that such material would not be helpful. Most groups did not feel that structured manuals, videotapes, professionally conducted educational lectures, professional workshops, and interactive workshops would be helpful.

After reviewing additional materials, the authors concluded that self-help groups are generally very successful in assisting newly diagnosed members and their families through the crisis following an initial diagnosis. Groups provide information and strategies related to (1) the culture of the specific disease, (2) coping with the full scope of problems related to the illness, and (3) achieving the highest possible quality of life. In addition, much of what self-help groups do is applicable to advanced disease stages. For example, groups generally help members:

- Learn how to negotiate the health care and other bureaucratic systems
- Understand the illness and treatment
- Make appropriate medical choices
- Evaluate the effects of medications and treatment
- Accept the impact of their illness
- Shift to a positive self-concept and identity
- Successfully change their relationships with family members, friends, and employment environments

In groups that do not have a specific process for dealing with members at the end of life, the empowerment approach of most peer-led groups can provide members with the experience and support they need to stay involved in major decisions related to the disease, the quality of their lives, and the circumstances of their death. In general, the following characteristics of self-help groups facilitate responses to loss and grief, to questions about the meaning of existence, and to changes in roles, which frequently arise in connection with a life-threatening illness.

- Members share a common condition, problem, symptom, or experience that transcends individual differences and creates a climate of acceptance, which is especially important at the end of life.
- Members govern themselves; they recognize that individual votes count as the group arrives at decisions through consensus. This experience of shared decision making can carry over into a wide variety of decisions at the end of life.
- Groups have a set of beliefs about how to deal with the illness, run meetings, and respond to individuals experiencing difficulty. When connected to national health or self-help organizations, the groups develop or receive succinct, authoritative health information sheets or packets. This material may contain information about and resources related to the terminal stages of the disease.
- Groups advocate self-reliance and self-responsibility, encouraging members to retain control of their lives. If members experience an existential conflict in the advanced stages of a disease, they are encouraged to realistically evaluate their expectations and responsibilities and to seek as much emotional satisfaction as possible in significant relationships.
- Groups advocate mutual aid among members. The "helper therapy principle" observed by Reissman (1984) and others states that the person helping benefits even more than the person helped. This can be particularly true at the end of life, when an individual sharing the condition of the dying person may feel more equipped than professionals or family members to maintain a compassionate, attentive, respectful attitude throughout the final stages. During the advanced stages of a disease, group members can communicate through visits to the home or health care institution or via the telephone or Internet.
- Groups provide hope throughout the disease stages. In the early stages, seeing a happy, active 10-year-old child with acute lymphoblastic leukemia can lift the gloom of parents of a newly diagnosed 5-year-old. At later stages, hope is provided by those successfully coping with multiple challenges; members learn to anticipate and rehearse possible future scenarios when they observe role models in later stages of illness. Members in advanced disease stages can provide hope for a high quality of life and for feeling in control until the end.
- Grassroots, autonomous self-help groups charge low or no fees and operate outside institutional restrictions. Professional services may at

times be insufficient or not available to members; however, groups are free to seek to help members find new treatments and services. While many groups welcome cooperative relations with professionals, they generally prefer to struggle financially to retain their autonomy rather than be absorbed by a bureaucratic organization. This spirit of independence is important to members at the end of life, who may need specific assistance in resisting dehumanizing bureaucratic policies and practices that currently dominate EOL care.

Models to Improve Self-Help Group Outreach at the End of Life

It is obvious from the above comments that the basic characteristics of self-help groups can benefit members in advanced disease stages, even without specific group guidelines for meeting the needs of these members. Families of deceased long-time self-help group members often make it a point to communicate to the group how much the phone calls, visits, balloons, and cards meant. A number of existing organizational models could be expanded to assist more life-threatening illness groups to improve the support they provide to members at the end of life, including the following:

Separate meetings for individuals in advanced disease stages. This model is currently used by groups with relatively large numbers of members in or anticipating the final stages of the disease. Test Positive Aware Network in Chicago offers daytime meetings for members too ill with AIDS to work. Y-Me for breast cancer and the Cancer Wellness Center also regularly provide separate sessions for members in advanced stages.

Breakout sessions within general meetings. In this scenario, the entire group meets for educational presentations and general fellowship, but different age groups (children, teens, adults), different family groups (parents, siblings), people at different disease stages (newly diagnosed, remission, active disease stage, advanced disease stage), or people interested in specific topics (self-care, natural healing techniques) meet separately to share the most relevant experiences and assistance for their particular circumstances.

Outreach activities serving members at the end of life. Self-help groups could create opportunities for online communication and visiting programs, be available during critical events pre-selected by the terminally ill member, and assist in connecting families to hospice- and institution-based programs.

In addition, a number of general developmental models could be adapted to guide self-help groups in assisting members at the end of life. For example, Patricia Fennell's Four-Phase Method for treating chronic and trauma syndromes is geared toward helping people come to terms with the impact of physical, behavioral, psychological, social, and interactive forces (all of which are in upheaval as death approaches). Fennel's four phases of chronic illness include: (1) trauma/crisis, (2) failure of stabilization/normalization, (3) existential conflict, and (4) integration. Similar to most stage models, including Elisabeth Kubler-Ross' stages of dying or Lawrence Kohlberg's stages of moral development, Fennell's approach is not sequential; phases may occur out of sequence or be repeated. For instance, a relapse can trigger the return of issues that arose in the initial crisis phase. If the self-help group provides members with the skills to successfully handle the initial crisis, these competencies can be called on to reduce the trauma associated with the relapse or terminal diagnosis.

Support for Achieving a Peaceful Death

We believe that self-help groups are capable of having a far more significant impact on members and families dealing with advanced disease stages than they do currently. The increasing attention to improving EOL care offers self-help groups a great opportunity to codify the various ways they do and could support members throughout the dying process. This new emphasis for self-help groups is particularly important because of the support it gives to the efforts of health professionals who are also struggling to provide better care for dying patients.

Simple techniques, some used for centuries, could be made available to self-help groups whose members are willing to be present at the moment of death. Many groups related to a life-threatening illness have a small number of individuals who are comfortable with this role, and with very little effort, this number could be greatly increased. Hannah Hedrick, a long-time yoga and t'ai chi chih instructor, coaches AIDS and cancer group members in techniques that facilitate spiritual growth before and during the dying process. In addition, if introduced during an early stage of the illness, breathing meditation and other activities can improve the quality of life of the ill person and the family in the years or months preceding death.

Creating a Peaceful Environment

Everyone choosing to support the dying person should focus on that person in order to respond intuitively and enter fully into the dying process. An individual particularly close to the dying person may be identified as the primary "guide."

Sound. Sound and music special to the individual, including singing, chanting, toning, and repeating of a mantra, can be used to improve the quality and comfort of the final hours or moments. Individuals can be asked in advance to select the music they would like to have played at the time of their death and during their memorial service.

Scent. Until recently, aromatherapy was ridiculed by skeptics attempting to discount the benefits of complementary health practices. But people with an illness have long requested smells they associate with pleasant memories, from cooking smells to baby powder to a favorite perfume.

Ritual. Prayer, meditation, and other spiritual techniques and rituals appropriate for the individual and family can enhance health and provide comfort in preparation for death and at the moment of death. Family rituals that can be conducted in low tones or in silence are especially appropriate.

Unfinished business and intuitive "messages." If there is time and if unfinished business (such as expressing gratitude, saying good-bye, or capturing a life review on video, on tape, or in writing) has not been resolved, the primary guide can help identify tasks and facilitate their accomplishment. And although it may sound strange to people who have not been present during a conscious death, sometimes the dying person will appear to speak or act through one of the participants. For example, Dr. Hedrick has been moved to say things that are very meaningful to a friend or family member, although she was unaware of the meaning. If a dying person appears to be struggling to wait for someone's arrival, the primary guide can assure the dying person that he or she is in intuitive communication with the loved one and need not "hold on" until the person arrives.

Peer Breathing Meditation—Release to Peace

After creating a peaceful environment, the primary guides can signal the beginning of the peer breathing meditation, based on well-established traditions and techniques. The benefits of meditation have been reported in scientific peer-review journals in recent years by physicians such as Herbert Benson, Dean Ornish, and Andrew Weil. Release of tension through moving or seated meditation, both involving breath awareness, can diminish physical pain, nausea, and shortness of breath and alleviate anxiety, anger, fear, and sleeplessness. Cross breathing or co-meditation, in which one person helps another to relax by breathing audibly, has been practiced for an estimated 3000 years. Richard Boerstler and Hulen Kornfeld (1995) have written extensively about the work they have conducted since 1979 to bring a modified co-meditation process into widespread practice. Their technique includes progressive muscle relaxation, a body scan, a sound sequence based on repeating "ahhhhh" (together and then by the facilitator alone), counting from 1 to 10 for 5 minutes to the rhythm of the recipient's breath, repetition of a word, words, or prayer chosen by the recipient, and conclusion of the session, which may include verbal cues for reducing tension.

Our experience with the peer breathing meditation began about 15 years ago. We found ourselves at the bedsides of people who had attended the Family Cancer Support Network's yoga, t'ai chi chih, and meditation sessions. Being with group members who knew these modalities led naturally to sharing meditative states at the moment of death. In 1987, Dr. Hedrick began to teach yoga, t'ai chi chih, and meditation two nights a week at an HIV/AIDS group. Many participants became regular meditators, and on several occasions, with no previous experience with a dying person, were perfectly comfortable participating in a "release-to-peace" group meditation. The power of the group process provided a cushion of comfort to family members and friends, who appreciated guidance in actively supporting the dying process of a loved one.

The processes vary somewhat, depending on the environment (intensive care, intermediate care, long-term care institution, home with hospice, home without hospice, nursing home hospice, institutional hospice) and the mental and physical state of the dying person. Various scenarios call for different accommodations; however, some elements are fairly constant: supportive physical position, sustained focus, gentle touch, following of the breath, body/mind/spirit connection, and request for and receipt of help and guidance.

Supportive physical position. After doing what can be done to establish a peaceful environment, the primary guide and supporters approach the dying person with respect and silently request permission to enter that person's space to support the dying process. Healing team members will usually move intuitively to a supportive position. Positions may change, with the primary guide moving from an initial position at the feet to higher points on the body as death approaches, ending around the heart or head during the last breath.

Sustained focus. The primary guide reminds supporters that if their focus shifts to their sense of loss or other issues, they should gently withdraw from close proximity to the dying person until they can regain a meditative focus.

Gentle touch. Depending on the mental and physical state of the dying person, the guide and supporters can do gentle "comfort" touching or hovering, staying in a state of absolute reverence and respect and being careful not to distract the dying person from the work involved in the active dying process. Sometimes the dying person is connected to so much equipment that only the feet and the head can be touched.

Following the breath. After establishing a sense of connection with the dying person, the guide tunes into and matches the sound and rhythm of that person's breath, even if the breath is harsh. It's as if the guide is assuming the effort of laboring for the breath, leaving the patient free to relax.

Body/mind/spirit connection. The above steps join all of the supporters in a meditative state with the dying person. An experienced primary guide can coach others in entering the space of the dying person. If family members persist in trying to get the dying person to respond to them, supporters may take them aside and comfort them.

Asking for help. Once the breathing of the guide and the dying person is synchronized and the connection between the two is deepened, the primary guide opens herself/himself to intuitive guidance, asking sincerely for help in where to be, what to say, and what to do to support the dying person. This state of receiving guidance continues throughout the dying process.

Accommodations for varied scenarios. Entering into a state of respectful communication with the dying person may visibly reduce agitation and distress. The guide or a supporter may further soothe the dying person by sitting or kneeling by the bedside in absolute silence and stillness, with the outside hand holding the dying person's hand and the other hand hovering above or lightly touching the upper abdomen or heart center. Those present at the deathbed need to guard against inappropriate stimulation that can distract the dying person. If active aspiration feels appropriate to diminish signs of physical and emotional agitation, it is generally best done by one person. If the process is prolonged and tiring, the guide may model soft breathing for the dying person by sitting at the head of the bed and cradling the dying person between his or her arms and legs.

Need for Resources and Training

Self-help groups are uniquely positioned to acquire and use tools to expand their outreach and better serve members at the end of life. Groups could seek external funding to conduct workshops geared to sensitize members about the need to provide support at the end of life. Self-help groups offer a laboratory for observing and learning about effective strategies for providing peer support at the end of life. Depending on the group, there are a number of options to serve members at the end of life. Groups would need to understand who attends their meetings, the needs of current members, and those of people who contact the group but decide the group does not meet their needs. By better understanding their constituency, groups could then address various options for meeting unresolved needs for the goals they target.

With modest support from various sources fueling current efforts to improve EOL care, self-help groups could provide members and families facing death with information and comfort to support them through the various stages of illness. These groups could be invaluable conduits for distributing consumer health education and actual assistance during the dying process. The burgeoning online support available on the Internet could be used even more effectively when mobility is difficult or when needing immediate communication from peers or professionals about whatever issues arise during the end of life, especially dealing with symptoms other than pain.

A real need exists for all members to be assisted in learning to handle emotional conflict, grief, and loss, with professional collaboration when desirable. We are seeking to learn about the risks and benefits of exposing self-help group members to EOL issues, how best to structure groups, and when it would be beneficial to bring together members at all stages of the disease. We hope to develop resources to help groups create and coordinate EOL programs. Please contact Dr. Daryl Isenberg of the Illinois Self-Help

Coalition, 773 481-8837, if you are interested in participating in a program of positive interventions to help self-help groups develop structures to more clearly understand and meet the needs of members and families preceding and following a death.

Resources

Boerstler, R and H Kornfeld. 1995. *Life to Death: Harmonizing the Transition.* Rochester, VT: Healing Arts Press.

Katz, AH, HL Hedrick, DH Isenberg, LM Thompson, TM Goodrich, and AH Kutscher. 1992. *Self-Help: Concepts and Applications.* Philadelphia, PA: The Charles Press.

Levine, S. 1987. *Healing into Life and Death.* New York, NY: Anchor Books/Doubleday.

Rinpoche, S. 1992. *The Tibetan Book of Living and Dying.* San Francisco, CA: HarperSan Francisco.

24

Patient Advocacy:
A Multidisciplinary Mandate

Dianne L. Locke, RN, MN, CS, and Anne H. Boyle, RN, PhD

Every health care provider involved in the care of the terminally ill is responsible for advocating quality-of-life interventions for such individuals. This means becoming an instrument for the vulnerable patient and acting on his or her behalf when needed, presenting the concerns, questions, and issues related to that patient. Advocacy mandates an approach that respects the values and professional commitments of all involved individuals, and advocates recognize that the patient's autonomy is meaningful and that appropriate care is first and foremost in everyone's mind (Quinn 1987).

Health care providers have long struggled with decisions about appropriate care for patients nearing death. Recently, there has been increased public demand for new standards governing end-of-life care, but despite these efforts, pain control is often not adequate, costly and unwarranted care is given, and a patient's preferences for the management of his or her care are often not recognized (SUPPORT Principal Investigators 1995).

Multidisciplinary Teams

In the not too distant past, physicians exercised complete control over the care plan for patients in any health care delivery system. The concept of "team" depended strictly upon the largesse and enlightenment of the individual physician or institution. The delivery systems themselves had little or no regard for the contributions and skills of other health care professionals. These situations were further complicated by the fact that patients and families often communicated differently to the physician than to the daily caregivers. Many nurses can relate stories of patients who say "I'm fine..." to the physician, but then verbalize a long litany of complaints and discomforts to the nurse, therapist, social worker, or other provider.

As society has begun to move away from the "scientific totalitarianism" described by Aldous Huxley in *Brave New World*, physicians are becoming more enlightened team leaders, seeking input from nonphysician health care team members. In fact, because of current forces within the health care delivery systems, physicians may not even be the team leaders. Managed care has severely limited physicians' time with patients, while other professions have skillfully demonstrated their unique contributions to patient care. Also, many physicians are pleased to have others share the challenges of such emotional situations as the end of life, while patients are recognizing that the entire team has nonmedical skills and interventions that contribute significantly to their care and outcome. Consequently, the various health care professions are increasingly being held accountable, by society and individuals, for their unique contributions to the health care team.

Challenges to Advocacy

However, even in a more enlightened environment, several limitations of advocacy and pitfalls for advocates still exist. Nonphysician team members may be hesitant to advocate for fear of reprisals from a system that does not value or facilitate open and equal dialogue between the health professions. Institutional procedures and policies may impede interdisciplinary communication patterns, eg, committees that are structured in such a way as to exclude the very professions that are in closest proximity to patients. Often, patients still are reluctant to "bother" or to be honest with their physicians, even though the 1990 Self-Determination Act names the patient as the captain of his or her team (Davison and Degner 1998). In addition, patients, their families, and other concerned individuals may change the concept of the desired care on a daily basis, with such decisions being based on the physical and emotional reserves available at that particular time.

Another serious difficulty that patient advocates face is societal ambiguity, as reflected in the mixed messages sent to caregivers. For example, in 1995, a physician in California was accused of murder for alleviating his patients' pain and discomfort with appropriate doses of narcotics. In Virginia in 1998, a physician was severely sanctioned for over-prescribing narcotics for his chronic pain patients. Yet, in 1999, a physician in Oregon was accused of failure to treat his lung cancer patients' pain and suffering with adequate medication. Nurses have been disciplined for interfering with the doctor/patient relationship by giving their patients additional information about treatment options (Quinn and Smith 1987) Yet, legal suits have resulted in judgments against nurses for failure to secure appropriate care. The patient advocate is clearly taking a risk. However, the principle of "double effect"—when the intervention aimed at the relief of symptoms may shorten the length of the patient's life, but the intent is relief of suffering and not to commit euthanasia—has been well-debated by society. Various professional organizations, including the American Nurses Association, have position statements that endorse the correctness and ethical appropriateness of such interventions (American Nurses Assn 1992).

Despite such constraining issues, all professions have a code or mandate of practice that can be, and often is, used as the standard by which individual professionals are evaluated. Relevant statements in the codes of some of the professions represented on the multidisciplinary health care team include:

Nurses: Nurses are "morally obligated to respect the individual needs and values of all persons"; "the nurses' primary commitment is to the patient's interests, even when there may be a conflict of interest among families, colleagues, or organizations" (American Nurses Assn 1997).

Pharmacists: Pharmacists "will consider the welfare of humanity and relief of human suffering [their] primary concerns"; "[they] will apply [their] knowledge, experience, and skills to the best of [their] ability to assure optimal drug therapy outcomes for the patients [they] serve"; "[they] will embrace and advocate change in the profession of pharmacy that improves patient care."

Social Workers: "The social worker's primary responsibility is to clients.... The social worker should make every effort to foster maximum self-determination on the part of clients" (National Association of Social Workers Code of Ethics).

Concerns and Arenas of Advocacy

Liaschenko (1995) describes the *concerns* of advocacy as links in a chain. The first link addresses the significance of the domain in which the need for advocacy arises. The greater the significance, the greater the possibility of harm imposed by the act, or lack of the act, of advocacy. Certainly, the domains of death, dying, and life quality are among the most significant. The second link states that the more vulnerable the individual requiring advocacy, the greater the opportunity to either advocate, or fail to advocate, for that individual. Patients facing their demise in a potentially suffering manner are highly vulnerable. The last link is about the potential for abuse of the power the advocate holds over the individual described in the first two links. Advocates must refrain from a paternalistic/maternalistic approach that does not include the values, wishes, strengths, and weaknesses of the cared-for individual. The links of advocacy—significant domain, vulnerability, and power—are clearly demonstrated in the example of an individual whose wishes involved no heroics and a health care provider who waved an endotracheal tube over his head, while berating him and his family about the need for immediate intervention.

Several *arenas* of advocacy are also depicted by Liaschenko (1995). The first is the physical arena, which entails working toward competent care of patients' physical needs. Poor nutrition, pain, dyspnea, and other symptoms may need to be accurately described, reported, and re-reported in order to achieve palliation. An often overlooked aspect of this arena is that of attending to environmental needs and navigating the health care system. Patients and families are often overwhelmed by bureaucracy and have no idea how to secure the care and services they need. They are frequently unaware of the services and care available to them. The second arena, the psychological arena, is full of opportunities for advocacy and controversy. Liaschenko (1995) describes this as the arena in which competent patients are supported and participate in informed treatment related to end-of-life issues and discussions. The final arena is that of "integrity of the self." The work in this arena consists of assisting dying individuals to identify their values and to use them in decision making. The challenge for providers arises when those values and decisions are different from their own. Practitioners must refrain from pushing their beliefs, however subtly, because this can unduly influence what patients say is the desired course of action (Hart et al 1998). In addition to being nonjudgmental and accepting, discussions of end-of-life plans and preferences require the ability to deal with painful and emotional issues.

Advocacy for COPD Patients at the End of Life

A formidable dilemma that clinicians face when dealing with chronic illnesses is determining when it is time to *care* rather than aim for a *cure*. In COPD especially, making this decision is more of an art than an exact science. Health care providers have certain measurements that may indicate that the terminal slide has begun, ie, FEV_1, frequency of hospitalization, or depression; however, these are in no way definitive markers. Many health care providers who have had patients that they believed were at death's door were surprised, instead, to see those patients go on to live many comfortable months. Caregivers inexperienced in dealing with end-stage COPD often encounter a great deal of discomfort providing palliative care to individuals who do not fit into the hospice mold of "6 months or less to live." However, Lynn and colleagues (1997) reported that patients facing the end of life preferred that their care be focused upon comfort, not cure. Therefore, securing a plan of care that includes such things as potent opiates for dyspnea, rehabilitation for enhanced activity tolerance, and home visits can present a real challenge to the patient and his or her caregivers.

Providing competent care to the person with COPD at the end of life requires an interdisciplinary team effort. The team must consist of all those who can contribute to the care of the patient, and members must work collaboratively. Aroskar (1998) defines the relationship between team members as "working together with mutual respect for the contributions and accountabilities of each profession to the shared goal of quality patient care." In order to facilitate these care teams, organizations must develop structures that empower autonomy of staff, while encouraging an atmosphere of openness to critical review (Hart et al 1998). Organizations can establish sessions that promote group problem solving so that an individual does not perceive himself or herself as the only advocate out on the proverbial shaky limb. Individual members of care teams also bear the responsibility of behaving as professionals who recognize the ultimate goal of quality patient care and autonomy. Listening to each other and learning from one another's experiences are vital to the process. Advocacy requires assertiveness, respect, flexibility, and participation. True commitment to the patient is not a spectator sport. Team members must explore their own values relating to end-of-life care and act as role models by expressing their advanced planning issues with their own families or surrogates. Every team member is responsible for establishing a climate that promotes the discussion of ethical issues and exploration of approaches to appropriate care. Individuals with COPD must clarify their values and do advanced life planning prior to becoming totally disabled and unable to participate in decision making. Most individuals are willing to discuss advanced care planning when the conversation is initiated by someone else (Sweibel and Cassel 1989). These discussions remove the burden of painful choices from the surrogate; the surrogate's role then becomes one of implementing the expressed wishes. This is a wonderful gift to give to loved ones.

Establishing rapport with patients through ongoing interaction enables advocates to understand the patients' desires. For example, when patients are reluctant to "bother" the physician, nonphysician advocates can assist in formulating questions and can support the patient by getting necessary information (Davison and Degner 1998). Advocates must also find out how much participation patients want to have in decision making. It is wrong to assume that all patients want to direct every decision made by the health care team. Advocates who make this assumption may be imposing their own autonomy values on the patients.

Patients at the end of life fear dying alone and with unremitting suffering. Uncertainty and fear are as much a part of suffering as pain and dyspnea (Cassell 1982). Care teams should be honest with patients, letting them know what to expect and providing the assurance that their symptoms can and will be managed.

Summary

Every health care provider, on assuming the role of a professional, is obligated to assist patients in identifying their values and interest in decision making, and to attain the care and control needed to make the end of life as quality an event as possible. As investigators of the SUPPORT study (1995) recommend, to provide appropriate care and to empower health care providers as advocates, health care professions and society must continue to refine the concept and practice of advance directives. Organizations and medical societies should continue to investigate the difficulties that physicians face when permitting patients to become the captains of their own teams. Health care systems must evaluate their weaknesses as user-friendly environments for patients and identify methods for modifying those weaknesses. And society as a whole must continue to explore the meaning of death in our lives and assist the health care professions in defining their roles in that process.

References

American Nurses Assn. 1992. Position statement on promotion of comfort and pain relief in dying patients. Washington, DC: American Nurses Assn.

American Nurses Assn and Center for Ethics and Human Rights. 1997. Code of ethics for nursing, draft #7. Washington, DC: Amer Nurses Assn/Ctr for Ethics and Human Rights.

Aroskar, MA. 1998. Ethical working relationships in patient care: challenges and possibilities. *Ethics for Nursing Practice*. 33(2):313-324.

Cassell, EJ. 1982. The nature of suffering and the goals of medicine. *New Eng J Med*. 306(11):639-645.

Davison, BJ and LF Degner. 1998. Promoting patient decision-making in life and death situations. *Seminars in Oncology Nursing*. 14(2):129-136.

Hart, G, P Yates, M Clinton, and C Windsor. 1998. Mediating conflict and control: practice challenges for nurses working in palliative care. *Intl J Nursing Studies*. 35(5):252-258.

Liaschenko, J. 1995. Ethics in the work of acting for patients. *Advances in Nursing Science*. 18:1-12.

Lynn, J, JM Teno, RS Phillips, AW Wu, N Desbiens, J Harrold, MT Claessens, N Wenger, B Kreling, and AF Connors for the SUPPORT Investigators. 1997. Perceptions by family members of the dying experience of older and seriously ill patients. *Ann Int Med*. 126(2):97-106.

Quinn, CA and MD Smith. 1987. *The Professional Commitment: Issues and Ethics in Nursing*, 77-101. Philadelphia: WB Saunders Co.

Stein, LI. 1967. The doctor-nurse game. *Arch General Psychiatry*. 16:699-703.

SUPPORT Principal Investigators. 1995. A controlled trial to improve care for seriously ill hospitalized patients. *JAMA*. 274(20):1591-1598.

Sweibel, NR and CK Cassel. 1989. Treatment choices at the end of life. *Gerontologist*. 29:615-621.

25

Last Acts: A National Coalition to Improve Care and Caring Near the End of Life

Victoria D. Weisfeld

- Only 41% of terminally ill patients report talking to their physicians about their prognosis.
- Physicians do not understand the cardiopulmonary resuscitation preferences of terminally ill patients 80% of the time.
- 50% of patients do not get the Do Not Resuscitate orders that they want.
- According to their families, 50% of patients are in pain in the last days of life.

Reported in 1995, these appalling situations were just some of the findings of a $28 million research study on end-of-life care funded by The Robert Wood Johnson Foundation (RWJF). The study, known as SUPPORT, and the widespread media coverage it received, rocked the health care community and served as a wake-up call that improvements were badly needed. For, despite the study's rigorous interventions to improve end-of-life care, postintervention results demonstrated no significant change in the way that dying people were treated.

Why was this and how could it be changed? RWJF responded by creating an ambitious, ongoing campaign to raise awareness and engage both health professionals and the public in making necessary changes. This campaign is named "Last Acts" for the acts that everyone can and should do—talking about tough issues, insisting on appropriate care, and educating others about needed changes—to ensure that the end of people's lives is one of comfort, dignity, and meaning. For its first 3 years, Last Acts was managed by RWJF. Campaign management is now being turned over to Partnership for Caring: America's Voices for the Dying. Partnership for Caring (PFC) staff have considerable substantive knowledge about the end-of-life field and, just as important, a history of collaboration and inclusiveness.

Goals and Structure of Last Acts

Last Acts has identified and given visibility to issues and initiatives, while inspiring others to action and providing the resources and tools for those actions to be effective. Since its inception, Last Acts has believed that improvements in end-of-life care depend on progress in

- improving provider-patient communication
- changing the culture of the medical care system so that it is more attentive to the needs of dying patients
- changing the American culture, which is so death-denying that progress is difficult

To accomplish these goals, Last Acts developed a unique structure that enables its work to proceed through the collaborative efforts of many diverse groups, with an emphasis on networking, relationship building, and encouragement of a movement in which "everyone" can participate.

The 3 main structural components of the Last Acts campaign are the partners, the committees, and the communications team. From the outset, Last Acts attracted a wide variety of organizations under the premise that everyone has a part to play in this change effort. The partners—some 500 organizations to date—have several roles. They are the "eyes and ears" of the campaign at both the community and national levels, bringing forward information about new developments and timely issues. They are a major resource for disseminating ideas and material from Last Acts to hundreds of their own members. They network with one another, creating momentum through the exchange of ideas and building on the successes of others.

At the first Last Acts national leadership conference, executives from 140 various organizations discussed what they believed to be the most important issues in end-of-life care and opportunities for action. Out of these discussions, Last Acts formed 11 committees to develop products (guidelines, conferences, reports, and tools) that would move the field forward. The 11 committee topics are: diversity, spirituality, family, workplace, professional education, institutional innovations, palliative care, financing, communications and policy, standards and guidelines, and evaluation and outcomes.

Three communications firms carry out the day-to-day work for Last Acts, each being responsible for either public policy, professional, or consumer issues. Within their respective areas, the firms track developments in the field, prepare articles and summaries for distribution to professionals and the public, network with leaders in the field and campaign partners, and facilitate the work of Last Acts committees.

Program Accomplishments

By using an array of communication strategies, Last Acts is credited with generating a collaborative atmosphere in the end-of-life field, forming much more powerful networking and synergy. In addition, from 1997 to 2000,

Last Acts has helped to develop a number of products that have yielded impressive results, including:

- 7 policy briefs, each mailed to more than 10,000 policymakers
- Consumer information advertising tied to an episode of the popular TV program, *ER*, that had end-of-life themes
- "Hollywood Initiative" activities that resulted in 4 prime time end-of-life story lines in 1999 and that exposed numerous entertainment writers and producers to Last Acts messages
- Thousands of brochures about loss and grieving that were distributed to consumers
- Medical and nursing textbook reviews that resulted in commitments from publishers to improve and expand end-of-life information
- An on-line journal, *Innovations in End-of-Life Care*, that has been read by more than 3000 professionals
- An award-winning Web site (www.lastacts.org) that receives almost 5,000 visits weekly

Future Plans for Last Acts

As the new national program office for Last Acts, PFC will provide management, leadership, and vision to the campaign, both expanding and consolidating its programs. Also, Last Acts will establish a National Advisory Committee and an Honorary Leadership Committee to guide and spearhead its efforts. Former First Lady Rosalynn Carter is the honorary chair of the campaign.

One of the program's expansion efforts will be to test the effectiveness of focusing on a theme or issue each year. This year, the theme will be "caregivers"—what can be done for and with family caregivers. All other activities will continue but, where appropriate, will incorporate caregiver issues and messages.

Last Acts will also involve its partners more actively. For example, "Affinity Conference Calls" will be designed around topics of special interest. These ongoing conference calls will enable partners to share ideas about important issues, such as hospice reimbursement, medical school curricula, or clergy involvement in the care of patients.

In addition, a national meeting will be held to receive and respond to the first annual "state of the nation" report on end-of-life care and caring. Partners and committee members will have an opportunity during the conference to engage in facilitated networking sessions to provide feedback and discuss information needs.

Last Acts programs will be more closely evaluated to ensure that desired outcomes are achieved. The ongoing evaluation will also enable the Last Acts teams to respond quickly if changes or adaptations are needed.

Finally, expansion efforts will also include special events, such as the reception and dinner on Capitol Hill to introduce policymakers and national leaders to the PBS television series, *On Our Own Terms: Bill Moyers on Dying in America*, and to encourage them to become involved in end-of-life issues.